The Complete
Home Guide
to Aromatherapy

The Complete Home Guide to Aromatherapy

Erich Keller

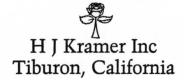

H J Kramer Inc
Tiburon, California

H J Kramer Inc.
P.O. Box 1082
Tiburon, CA 94920

Editor: Nancy Grimley Carleton
Cover Art and Design: Spectra Media
Composition: Classic Typography
Book Production: Schuettge & Carleton
Manufactured in the United States of America
10 9 8 7 6 5 4 3

Library of Congress Cataloging-in-Publication Data

Keller, Erich.
    The complete home guide to aromatherapy / Erich Keller.
        p. cm.
    Includes bibliographical references.
    ISBN 0–915811–36–7
    1. Aromatherapy. I. Title.
RM666,A68K45   1991
615′.321 — dc20   91–52841
                                                            CIP

To Our Readers

The books we publish
are our contribution to
an emerging world based on
cooperation rather than on competition,
on affirmation of the human spirit rather
than on self-doubt, and on the certainty
that all humanity is connected.
Our goal is to touch as many
lives as possible with a
message of hope for
a better world.

Hal and Linda Kramer, Publishers

Contents

Introduction

Six years ago, my girlfriend came home and showed me some amber-colored bottles filled with strongly smelling oils. From the moment I opened these bottles and smelled the pure, concentrated fragrance of flowers and plants, my life changed dramatically. I still remember the mystifying sensation I experienced with my first whiff of jasmine. Everything stopped for a moment, I forgot where I was, and I simply became the sense of smell.

Until that time, I had never been very interested in scents. Of course, I preferred some smells and disliked others, but, as is the case for most people, this sense remained in the background.

On that night, however, I felt as if I were entering and dissolving into the aromas. I felt my consciousness expand. I could never have imagined what was going to happen to me after this first ecstatic encounter with essential oils.

During the following days, I visited my girlfriend in her scent shop and spent time opening all the bottles, smelling and experiencing each unique essential oil. I purchased an aroma lamp, and from then on my home was always filled with the enchanting aromas of essential oils.

I prepared my first aromatic bath, using a blend of sandalwood, cypress, and vanilla, which provided a feast for my newly awakened senses. As I savored this bath, I became deeply relaxed; I had never before felt so blissful. This experience awakened something deep inside me. I felt as if I had found a long lost friend. After a few more days spent inquiring into the practical application of aromatherapy, I blended my first perfume, using my favorite scents. This perfume was such a success that I found I wanted to know everything there was to know about essential oils, and I studiously read the few books I could find. I began to create my own face creams, massage oils, hair conditioners, and shampoos.

Whenever people passed me in the street, I immediately caught the essence of their perfumes. While walking in nature, I paid much more attention to the flowers and plants. I picked leaves and rubbed them, trying to become familiar with their fragrance. I felt much more connected to the natural world and discovered a deeper respect for the living things surrounding me. The herbs I used in the kitchen, the fruit on the table, and the flowers in my garden all took on a new meaning as I began to find out about their therapeutic and healing properties.

A new kind of love arose in me—a deep love toward nature, and existence. I became thankful for all of the trees, plants, and herbs that offer us their life energy in the form of essential oils. I realized the amazing potential of smell to heal and transform, and I decided to take the time to learn how to tune into it and use it. I paid much more attention to my body and studied how the healing properties of the essential oils could help me. I am happy to say that I have not needed to take any pharmaceutical medicine since the day I became acquainted with the healing properties of aromatherapy.

Wherever I travel, I take along my collection of essential oils. Whenever I enter a sterile hotel room, I immediately take out my aroma lamp and fill the room with comforting, pleasant smells. While flying in an airplane, I prevent my typical clogged nose and mild headache with a dry inhalation of peppermint oil, and relax with a few drops of lavender oil on my tissue. Of course, my fellow passengers are often intrigued by both my actions and the unusual smells circulating about the plane, and they want to have a go at it, too! When I traveled in India, I wore a special blend of skin oil to ward off the hungry mosquitoes, and I swallowed a few drops of oil daily to defend myself against the infamous intestinal disruptions of that teeming subcontinent.

After my trip to India, I was given the chance to work at the very scent shop that had originally launched me on my aromatic path, and I eagerly jumped in. This new role seemed second nature to me, as if I already knew all I needed to know deep inside myself. I had a wonderful time advising people, knowing that I really was offering them something valuable. I entered into the never-ending process of reading, studying, and developing my expertise. Now, whenever I am working with essential oils and aromatherapy through treating, healing, or advising, I feel supported by life, and events flow smoothly and easily. I decided to write this book to share both my experiences and the joy of working and living with essential oils.

The purpose of this book is to enable you to know and understand the properties of essential oils and the basics of aromatherapy—healing with aromas. With this knowledge, you will be able to help, heal, and care for your body, your mind, and your spirit.

Your journey to the land of scents will begin with a look at the history of the uses of essences. You will see how scents determine your reactions and influence your emotions. Later, you will learn the practical applications of aromatherapy and study each essential oil, and its qualities and uses. You will finish your journey with an index of symptoms and treatments, which will enable you to find the right essential oil for every situation. I hope that soon you will find as much joy as I have in becoming an aromatherapist.

1
A History of Healing With Essences

The first human beings had a very distinct sense of smell, which was essential for their survival and reproduction. A long time before humans were able to think, the part of the brain that contains the sense of smell, called the limbic system, was already developed. The scents of edible plants, berries, fruits, mushrooms, potable water, and edible meat provided an important means of identification in the search for appropriate food and water. Smell even helped determine the choice of a sexual mate at the right time.

After the discovery of fire, early humans used branches, dry grass, and plants as fuel. In this way, they must have discovered the effects of different scents, such as sleepiness, excitement, relaxation, or joy. In addition, the ingestion of plants, fruit, and berries caused specific bodily reactions. Early humans also watched animals selecting particular plants for their basic nutritional qualities and to treat sickness.

Emulating animals and following their own senses, however, did not answer the question "Why is this so?" So, with increasing intelligence, human beings began to search for the cause and source of their reactions to particular plants and fruits. This was the beginning of the practice of healing with herbs, which over time led to healing with scents.

The art of aromatherapy—healing with scents— has its basis in healing methods that existed long before essential oils were known.

Lying beneath the 60,000-year-old skeleton of a man in what is now modern-day Iraq, researchers found a vessel containing the pollen of the healing herbs and flowers growing in that area. This man might have been a botanist, healer, or shaman. In China, as far back as 2000 B.C., healing with herbs was well known and widely practiced. One healing manual listed more than eight thousand recipes. A verse of the ancient religious scripture the Indian Rigveda (dated approximately 2000 B.C.) reads: "Come, beloved plant, and heal this patient for me."

The Egyptians considered scents and essences the most effective methods of healing. They believed that scents had been given to humanity by the gods for precisely this reason. The rarest and most valuable scents were reserved for the Egyptian kings, or pharaohs. In some pharaohs' gardens, the ponds contained rose-scented water. When the pharaohs died, their bodies were treated with the resin of the conifer (needle tree) to prevent the destructive effects of bacteria on the body. The fabric in which the bodies were wrapped contained frankincense, myrrh, cedarwood, and other balsamic resins and oils. In this way, the pharaoh could start his journey into another world and another life. The results of these treatments became evident thousands of years later as archaeologists discovered the mummies in the burial chambers of the pyramids. The bodies of the pharaohs were well preserved, and a famous psychic could still feel their energy lingering around. In the burial chamber of King Amon, one researcher found an airtight container of essences that had retained their scents for over 3,500 years!

Kings weren't the only ones to treat themselves with essences. Common people used a deodorant comprised of myrrh, frankincense, rosemary, and thyme. These essential oils were blended with a fatty substance, and formed into a small cone. The cone was placed under the clothing, and it gradually melted during the heat of the day. Today, we also know about the antiseptic, stimulating, and deodorizing effects of these oils. Yet the Egyptians were working with oils five thousand years ago, while most of the world was still in the darkness of precivilization.

In Babylon of 2000 B.C., we again hear of kings receiving massages with essential oils and taking scented baths. They used the essences of the local plants, trees, and herbs: cedarwood, cypress, myrrh, frankincense, galbanum, rose, jasmine, and so forth. Kings were able to enjoy these essences in a more frivolous way than the general population, who used essential oils and their scents mainly to treat medical disorders.

In approximately 1000 B.C., the process of distillation in Persia signaled a significant step forward in aromatherapy. Distillation made it possible to obtain essential oils from plants without the impurities that the previous method of extraction had entailed.

A Greek, Theophrastus, wrote a book entitled

"On Scents," which may well be the first book on aromatherapy. The Arabs were responsible for the spread of Asian scents and the knowledge of their uses, as they were the main traders of scents and other commodities between East and West. They imported musk from Tibet, sandalwood from India, and camphor from China, and traded these with Western empires.

In the first century B.C. and the first century A.D., the Romans brought back many exotic things from their war campaigns, and with each new military advance, they introduced these new treasures to cities throughout the Old World. Thus, the Roman Empire's wealthy and powerful enjoyed scented baths and massages, and the art of bathing was brought to the cities of Europe. Romans were also the first to produce fine cosmetics. For example, "cold cream" was first manufactured by a man named Galen, and his basic recipe is still used by modern cosmetics factories with just a little more refinement and the addition of synthetic ingredients. In ancient Rome, aromatherapy and cosmetics were divided into two different disciplines for the first time.

The Sufis, an Eastern religious sect, also worked with scents. They used them for spiritual exercises, enhancing their meditations with particular scents. The Sufis believed that humans have several vibrational bodies and that each should be treated with different scents. This old knowledge is well worth incorporating into our modern approach to healing.

Eventually, extensive trade flourished between the continents. The alchemists of Europe came to know about foreign herbs, plants, resins, and essences.

They used them to fight viruses during the times of the horrifying and far-reaching plagues. The resins of pine, cedarwood, and cypress were burned in the streets and in hospitals. Sage and thyme were burned in hospital rooms. Miraculously, many people working with these plants in storehouses and in the field, and especially the alchemists, did not get the plague. The reason for this "miracle" was that they were saved by the scent of the herbs and the essential oils with which they were working.

In the sixteenth century, an Englishman, Nicholas Culpeper, did extensive research on the healing and stimulating properties of plants, herbs, and essences. Culpeper's work and his publications spread and increased the knowledge and use of this healing method in Europe. To this day, Culpeper's work remains an instructive, fascinating collection of information and recipes.

In the twentieth century, the French chemist Gattefosse researched perfumes and cosmetics. In his hometown of Grasse, located in Provence, he rediscovered the healing properties of essential oils. This process began when he burned his hand while doing a test. He put his hand into a container of lavender oil, as he already knew of the healing properties of this essence. Surprisingly, no blisters appeared, the hand healed quickly, and no scars remained. This event led him to undertake research on the properties of essential oils. In 1928, he published his first book on the subject, and coined the term "aromatherapy."

Another Frenchman, Dr. Jean Valnet, was inspired

by Gattefosse's publications. He had already been working with herbs and had been successful in healing his patients with natural medicine. He then studied the properties of essential oils and soon began to treat patients solely with essences and herbs. He wrote one of the classic books in the field of aromatherapy, *The Handbook of Aromatherapy.*

At the same time, the French biochemist Madame Maury enriched the new "old" knowledge by developing information on the cosmetic and medical effects of essential oils.

The city of Grasse in the south of France is still the world's trade and production center of essential oils and other scented items for the cosmetic industry. Although there are other places where essential oils are produced using advanced, high-tech methods, Grasse remains the birthplace of modern aromatherapy, a great source of materials, and a place well worth visiting.

Today, you can find natural essential oils and other scented items such as bath oils, body oils, and facial cosmetics in body-care shops, scent shops, and in natural food stores. These precious essences give you natural agents to strengthen and heal your body and create a unity of mind and body. Given the stresses of modern life and the detrimental influences of our industrial environment, the benefits of essential oils are a valuable gift.

2
What Is the Sense of Smell?

After spending time in the polluted air of any modern city, or after shopping in big malls with their artificial air and scents, we often feel dizzy or experience a headache. Our breathing is shallow. Yet if we leave the city and take a walk in a pine forest, slowly our headache fades away, and we feel good again. We breathe deeply, and we feel alive again.

When we engage in shallow breathing, we get less oxygen, which our brain needs for its optimal functioning, and a feeling of tension and fear is created.

The scent of pine and fir trees enhances and deepens breathing. This ignites a chain reaction of processes in the body and emotions. To see how this works, take a moment to notice your breath without changing it. Then imagine that you are walking through a forest with a soft breeze of fresh air blowing. The air smells of firs, pines, grass, and flowers. How do you feel and breathe now?

Often upon entering a hospital ward, our breathing becomes shallow, unconsciously creating defensive feelings. Perhaps we feel we want to leave the hospital as soon as possible. The scent of a sick person—the smell of disease evaporating through the sweat—is totally different from the scent of a healthy person.

We all recognize these scents. Even without smelling the specific scent of sickness, you may find you can pick up the vibrations of disease. Psychics can discern these vibrations, which help them to determine the location and origin of illness. We are all psychic, although this capacity is better developed in some than in others, and our subconscious tells us when an illness is present. Today, scientists explain that the molecules comprising scent have specific vibrations that are recognized by the olfactory sense. Due to these vibrations, we feel uncomfortable in a hospital; we experience an instinctive, defensive reaction signaling us to leave or to be careful. This is our body's way of protecting us from possible infection or disease. Conversely, if we are ill, the flowers others bring to cheer us up also have the ability to heal us through their scent.

When walking in nature past blossoming bushes and flowers, or even when passing flowers in a vase, we often take a flower carefully in our hand to sniff it. As we do this, we are judging the scent, deciding whether we like it, and also whether we recognize it. Many processes are taking place in our brain, mainly in the limbic system. The scent is received as a bit of information and checked against previous information regarding scents. If we find an applicable bit of information, we can give the scent a name. Remembrances of emotions connected with this scent—happenings, places, and people—may flash in our memory. Through the linked information in our memory, we judge the particular scent as appealing or unappealing.

The stimulating influences of scents affect us very quickly. For example, smell a real, scented rose. Who does not know this joyful, relaxing aroma? Whose face does not break into a smile when inhaling this scent? The heart opens and expands. This is a very simple example of how scents affect our feelings.

Take a moment to imagine you are passing a bakery in the early morning. Do you feel hungry? Is saliva gathering in your mouth? Or imagine the scent of your favorite meal. Can you feel the changes in your body? On the other hand, smelling food over a long period makes us lose our appetite. In fact, this can serve as a way to eat less and lose weight.

In becoming aware of the aroma of food and drink, we begin the process of digestion. If there is not enough food in our stomach, we may become hungry from the smell. The scents of certain foods always seem to trigger the urge to eat. The process of digestion starts with the scent, saliva gathers in the mouth, and the composition and amount of acid in the stomach changes according to the food smelled.

If you have the flu or a cold, you cannot smell very well, and thus you are not likely to have much appetite. At these times, nothing tastes very good because the bridges between the senses have been disconnected. By the way, your sense of taste knows only sweet, salty, sour, and bitter. The rest of the pleasure of eating, and the fine nuances of taste, are formed by the sense of smell. Without scent, it would not matter what you ate, as it would all taste pretty much the same!

We all know the feeling of not liking somebody's

smell. We may say, "I can't stand this person." We may have difficulty working or getting along with that person. The real reason may be the person's smell. Each person has an individual smell, which changes slightly if that person is healthy, sick, angry, in love, aggressive, or joyful.

These aromatic messages are sent by everyone and are received by everyone. You can imagine how much scent information is received in a crowded place, a packed elevator, a cinema, a theater, a sports arena, or a shopping mall. You can also get a sense of how this rush of information can affect your emotions. Just imagine how you would react if you were in a fearful or aggressive crowd.

We can all give ourselves a scent "mask" by using perfume and thus altering our influence on others by smelling "fresh," "pleasant," "sexy," or "male." This will also affect us, changing our own emotions quite markedly. Scent is often the unconscious reason we like certain people, why we are drawn to them. While some people find the scent of another person's sweat sexy, sweat or perspiration actually evaporates the scents of sexual hormones, or pheromones, which can trigger our sexual desire. The scent of sex is an important part of desire, choice of partner, and choreography of the act itself.

We continuously smell everything that surrounds us — our car, our house, our city, our part of the country. Everything has its own individual scent. Familiar scents make us feel comfortable. We will never feel at home in a house that has a scent we don't like. Similarly, there is a big difference between living in a Western city and an Asian city, with its scents that are often too strong for our conditioned Western noses. Our sense of smell is trained from our very first breath, and our olfactory sense notices unpleasant odors more profoundly than pleasant ones, perhaps as a way to warn us that something is rotten, indigestible, unhealthy, or poisoned.

Scent is a molecule that disconnects itself from its carrier and drifts in the air. The nose is the organ of smell. In the upper part of the nose is a mucous membrane with approximately ten million odor-receptor cells and sixty million cilia, which can catch and identify any scent at any time. The cilia—tiny hairs—are extensions of the actual nerve cells. Unlike all other senses, here the nerve system is directly exposed to its source of stimulation. The cilia, as neurons, lead directly to the olfactory bulb in the brain. This explains the immediate effect of scents on the nervous system.

The science of the sense of smell is not fully developed yet, and there are still questions about how it really works. For example, one theory states that there are five different types of odor-receptor cells functioning like a lock. When scent molecules that have the shape of a certain "key" arrive, they fit into the corresponding "lock." The scent message is then passed along, and a particular scent's information is delivered to the brain. According to this theory, one set of locks would only receive molecules with a peppermint type of smell. Others would receive floral, musky, camphorlike, or ethereal scent molecules. Two additional "locks" are designated for pungent and putrid odors.

Another theory concentrates on the fact that odor molecules also absorb infrared radiation. Therefore, the nose might function like a spectroscope with the ability to analyze the molecules.

Finally, there is the theory of vibration, which proposes that every molecule has an individual rate of vibration that will be recognized by the neurons of the olfactory sense. If you consider your whole being as a vibrational unit, your senses recognize the vibrations of any form—even the vibrations of colors. This has actually been tested and proven with people who are able to "feel" colors with their tactile sense. This explains why your skin is sensitive when interacting with scented liquids or essential oils.

Each of these theories explains how the olfactory sense can discern a particular scent from a wide range of possibilities.

Let us continue exploring the process of smell. We receive a scent molecule, and its information is sent via the nerves to the olfactory epithelium (part of the limbic system) in the brain. The interpretation of the odor starts here and is sent from the limbic system to the thinking part of the brain. The limbic system is the oldest part of your brain, storing the information about every scent you have ever smelled. Via the nervous system and the hormones, it gives instructions on how to react to various stimuli. It also compares the information with its previously stored data concerning this scent.

Since the limbic system is also the seat ɩ memory, comparisons and connections between current odors and ones experienced in the past are made here.

This is why, for example, we may have a pleasant reaction to someone whose scent consciously or unconsciously reminds us of a loved one. Or, conversely, we may experience an aversion to a particular odor associated with something unpleasant in our past.

Our ability to learn and our capacity for sympathy is also located in the limbic system. The feelings of sympathy and antipathy are, as mentioned earlier, often connected with a person's body smell. In addition, the effects of essential oils on one's sexuality are caused by the relationship of this part of the brain with the hypothalamus, which communicates with the sex glands. Pheromones, which can trigger sexual desire when we smell them, are found in the body's sweat, urine, vaginal secretions, and saliva. In a later chapter, we will take a look at the abilities of certain scents to stimulate sexuality.

The limbic system also houses the basis for creativity, inspiration, and all autonomic life processes (breathing, digestion, excretion, heart function, hormones, immune system, and so forth). Scents affect each of these areas, too, and cause the body's systems and organs to react. Some scents enhance our memory, concentration, and thinking. Some can result in a clear mind. And others can make us calm, relaxed, and peaceful. From my experience, creativity is also enhanced by the scents a particular person likes the best. Search for the scents you find most pleasing; these will be the most important for your creative expression.

Scents have a short life. They lose their energy very quickly once dispersed into the air. Once inhaled, a scent will fade away after a few seconds if new molecules are not forthcoming. In addition, the olfactory neurons also tire quickly. For this reason, you cannot continuously smell a scent for a lengthy period of time. Broadly speaking, you will not smell the rose garden while you are sitting in the middle of it. You will recognize only the first molecules of scent and then grow accustomed to them. It should also be noted that a strong scent does not necessarily have a greater effect than a weaker one. A gentle whiff of a scent can cause the same reaction in the nervous system as a highly concentrated dose.

Since scents, including those in the form of essential oils, affect our bodies and emotions in so many ways, aromatherapy is a logical method for healing the body, the mind, and the spirit.

Some aromatherapists are even quite successful working on their clients' energy centers (chakras) with essential oils. Using scents to calm and relax people can lead to their spiritual growth, since calm people can more easily hear the messages of their soul and heart. Because scents can lift us up and allow a space for meditation, they are a tremendous aid to self-discovery.

These natural healers, the essential oils, contain the spirit of the plants, trees, fruit, and flowers from which they are derived. Their life force makes them totally different from synthetic drugs, which have no life force. In aromatherapy, the spirits of humans and plants meet. This is the most subtle aspect of aromatherapy. You can chemically create similar structures, but these will never contain life force. Synthetic drugs do not have those vibrations. In aromatherapy, we do not use the essences of minerals, as they are "dead" or "stuck" energy, or they have a very low vibration. In aromatherapy, we also never use essences from animal glands, as they can carry the vibrations of the suffering of the animals from which they are derived.

Knowledge about the power and effect of scents is not confined to aromatherapists only. Many household items and consumer products have been scented by the manufacturers in order to entice us to buy them. Some common examples are imitation leather jackets, which are scented with the aroma of real leather; cars smelling of musk, amber, or woody scents; magazines with scented perfume advertisements; frozen foods scented to give you the feeling that you are eating fresh food; and so forth. The next time you walk through a big shopping center, notice the multitude of artificial scents.

Once you sharpen your olfactory senses through aromatherapy, you will be able to tell the difference between natural and unnatural scents and begin to make the choices in your life to bring about better health and more vital spirit.

3

A Basic Guide to Essential Oils

Obtaining Essential Oils

A variety of methods are used to obtain essential oils from whole plants, leaves, blossoms, roots, barks, resins, or fruit peels. The basic process is to break the cell's wall, thereby releasing the essential oil.

Method 1: Maceration

In maceration, the blossoms are dipped into hot oil until the walls of the cells break apart and the hot oil absorbs the essence. Later, the oil and the essence are separated. This is an old-fashioned and expensive method rarely used today.

Method 2: Pressing

Essences of citrus fruits, such as oranges, lemons, grapefruits, and tangerines, are obtained by pressing the unpolluted, natural peels of the fruit. This type of essence is of high quality and suitable for internal use.

Method 3: Distillation

Distillation, one of the most basic methods, uses either hot water or steam to separate the essence from the plant. At a certain temperature, the cell's wall breaks and the essence evaporates. During the cooling process, the essence becomes a liquid again and can be bottled. The remaining water is a useful ingredient for cosmetics. Today, pure steam distillation is the most popular method for obtaining large amounts of essences in an industrial process, and it is only appropriate for plants with a large amount of essences— for example, peppermint. The superheated steam process is relatively inexpensive, which is reflected in the prices of the essences obtained in this fashion. These essences are of high quality, pure, and suitable for internal use.

Method 4: Extraction

Extraction is reserved for plants with a low concentration of essential oils (for example, jasmine), or with mostly resinous constituents. These oils usually have a finer fragrance. Two methods are used to extract the essential oils.

In the first, the blossoms are spread on perforated metal sheets and washed continuously with the same water until all essential oils are dissolved. Afterward, the essential oils are separated from the water by distillation.

In the second method, the essential oils of some flowers are isolated with a solvent, such as petrol ether. After the solvent has evaporated, a paste remains, called *essence concrete*. This paste also contains waxes and chlorophyll, and is only partly soluble in alcohol. The paste is mixed with alcohol, heated to 120 degrees Fahrenheit, cooled again, and filtered.

The remaining alcohol is removed through evaporation. Finally, an oily residue remains, called *essence absolute.* It is totally soluble in alcohol. This is a high-cost process, which is, of course, reflected in the price of the essential oils produced in this fashion.

Today, extractions are also made using carbon dioxide, a liquid gas. This allows the work to be done with low temperatures, which in turn preserves the quality of very fragile fragrances such as lily of the valley.

The essential oils obtained by extraction using the second method—called *essences absolutes,* or absolute oils—are not suitable for internal use as they always contain residues of the solvents.

Method 5: Enfleurage

Enfleurage is a very old, traditional method formerly used to obtain fine fragrances but today used only to isolate the oil of tuberose. The blossoms are spread on metal sheets with animal fats or in oil-soaked fabric, and continuously replaced with new blossoms until the fats or oils are totally enriched with essential oils. This process can take up to three weeks. By adding alcohol and with further distillation, the essential oils can be separated from the fat or oil. If not separated, the fats or oils are used for cosmetics such as body oils, creams, and pomades. They are expensive creams of high quality, called *huiles françaises.* The essential oils obtained in this manner are called *essences absolutes,* or absolute oils. They are not suitable for internal use.

You can understand why absolute oils are very expensive. A large number of flowers are needed to produce a small amount of essential oil. It takes one thousand pounds of petals to make approximately two pounds (thirty-two ounces) of rose oil! To avoid the high prices of true, natural, and pure absolute oil, trading companies often offer absolute oils diluted with ninety percent vegetable oil. This does not affect or damage the healing properties, and the scent is still strong since these oils are very highly concentrated.

General Properties of Essential Oils

Essential oils vary in consistency. Rose oil is very thick, and lavender oil is as thin as water. All are highly concentrated, with absolute oils having the highest concentration. They evaporate quickly if exposed to air. Evaporation times vary. Essential oils do not always smell like the original plant or blossom, and therefore it's easy to get confused by the smell. The intensity of the scent is individual. See the appendix at the end of the book for specific rates of intensity and evaporation.

Although essential oils are *called* oils, they are not really oils. They are not fatty and can be dissolved with fats and other substances.

Essential oils vary in color from green (rose, bergamot), to blue (German blue chamomile), to brown (jasmine), to red (myrrh). The oil's color lends the first hints about which healing properties you can expect. For example, the blue of German blue chamomile is a cooling color, and it is the opposite of red, a fiery, burning color. German blue chamomile is used for skin inflammations that appear red.

Essential oils can dye fabric, and they are flammable. If you squeeze an orange peel over a candle, you can see sparks as the essential oil burns.

Storage

Essential oils should be stored in amber-colored glass bottles in a cool place, as both sun rays and warmth can damage their properties. Stored properly, most essential oils will keep their properties for many years, except for citrus oils, which can only be kept for six months. Immediately after use, close the bottles tightly to prevent any evaporation. Massage oil or body-oil blends should also be stored in amber-colored bottles. I do not recommend using plastic containers, as the substances in the plastic, when combined with the essential oil, can cause a chemical reaction that damages the essence.

Basic Use of Essential Oils

Except in a few rare cases, most oils should not be applied undiluted to the skin. Any application of undiluted essential oils into the eyes is very hazardous. They should also not be applied undiluted on any mucous membrane or on the genitals. To dilute essential oils, you can use any vegetable oil, whipped cream, honey, alcohol, or liquid soap. For internal use, essential oils should be diluted with a lot of water and some honey and mixed vigorously. A true, pure essential oil will never dissolve by itself.

Blending

Essential oils can be blended to enhance their properties or to create a more pleasant scent. Lavender generally boosts the healing properties of other oils. Clove tends to boost the general scent of a blend. Bergamot is a good balancer of scents. It also can be used to cover up unpleasant scents of oils that you might need to cure yourself.

It is important to blend oils that possess the same character. To hinder fast evaporation, such as in an aroma lamp or perfume, you can blend quickly evaporating oils with slower ones. Although blending essential oils has its place, a large quantity of essential oil or a blend of many different oils does not have more beneficial effects than a small quantity of one appropriate oil.

Most essential oils are safe, but some can cause undesired effects or poisoning if used in overdose. Chapter 17 describes all the essential oils, along with any side effects they might produce. Remember to stick to the amounts mentioned in the recipes given in this book.

Quality and Price

Quality is an important consideration when purchasing and using essential oils, as you want to make sure you're using a natural, pure, and true healing agent and essence. Only genuine essential oils can guarantee the expected effects. Look for products that guarantee genuine, pure, and natural oils. Oils obtained from organically grown plants are more expensive, but their higher quality often makes them worth the price.

To give an example of the quality and price of essential oils, let us look at jasmine oil. Millions of blossoms are needed to obtain one pound of pure oil of jasmine. The plant itself does not contain much essential oil. The blossoms are harvested during the early morning at sunrise, as the essential oil gathers in the blossom at night. During the day, the oil moves to the stalks and leaves, but these cannot be harvested, because that would destroy the plant. Once the blossoms are harvested, the process of production is costly. An inexpensive oil of jasmine can never be genuine, pure, and authentic.

If you look around in the shops or in catalogs, you will find the best prices for essential oils. Bear in mind, however, that all over the world there are suppliers whose goal is to make as much profit as possible by using the minimum amount of pure essential oil. They extend the oil with similar oils, vegetable oils, and alcohol, or they may offer synthetic oils. The synthetics have no healing properties at all. Although they smell good, your olfactory sense does not recognize them as healing agents. You will experience none of the effects you might expect, since these substances have no life force. They simply smell nice.

Diluted oils do not have the total healing properties of pure oils. You can never be sure which substances the dilution contains unless the label states that an absolute oil is diluted with a high-quality vegetable oil.

Another method for extending essential oils is the use of toxic solubles to get more essential oils from the plants, but such solubles may remain even after distillation, making an inexpensive essence a poor bargain.

Terminology

What do the terms "pure, natural, and complete," and "genuine and authentic," really mean? "Pure, natural, and complete" means that no vegetable oils, synthetic material, or other essential oils have been added nor have any substances been taken out. Also, such oils are not decolorized. "Genuine and authentic" means that the oil is pure, natural, and complete and has been carefully distilled, never redistilled, to assure maximum authenticity.

Another term you should be familiar with is "adulterated." Adulterated oils are produced for two main reasons. First, to improve or change the scent of an oil, the similar-smelling substances of another oil may be added. For example, a rose oil may be altered with other types of rose oils or geranium oil. Second, the main substance of an oil may be isolated, leaving an oil with only a few of the originally existing substances. For example, eucalyptol, the main substance of eucalyptus or cajeput, may be isolated to provide an oil that only has this substance. Otherwise, such natural substances are added to an oil to enrich its healing power. But both scientists and therapists know that the whole, genuine oil has more healing power than the adulterated.

The term "perfume oil" refers to an impure, extended, or synthetic oil.

Quality Tests

There are a number of tests that can help you detect impure falsifications of essential oils.

(1) Put a drop of the oil on your finger. If it feels greasy, the essence was probably extended with vegetable oil.

(2) Put a drop of the oil in water. Essential oils do not mix with water! If the drop dissolves, or if it produces a milky or opaque solution, then the oil contains emulsifiers. Such oils are often produced for cosmetic and industrial uses.

(3) Put a drop of the oil on a blank piece of white paper. After the oil evaporates, it should leave no residue. If you see an oily stain, then the oil has been extended.

(4) Smell the oil. If you detect a whiff of alcohol, then the oil has been extended with ethyl alcohol. Quite naturally, after a while spent sniffing essential oils you soon will be able to detect falsifications.

Price and Value

As stated earlier, price is the basic guideline for the value of an essential oil. Be especially careful when an oil is very cheap. Unfortunately, I cannot give you a definitive price list, since prices vary a great deal among retail shops and big trading companies. They are also dependent upon the world economic situation as well as on the harvests in various countries. Also, if there is a high demand for essential oils, the price will generally be higher.

Essential oils are little treasures. They contain

the spirit and life energy of a particular being in the plant realm. They can help and strengthen us in a natural and pure manner. However, the life on our world is finite. Industrial and urban sprawl are eating up the open spaces. Our air, water, and soil are constantly being exposed to toxins. These factors determine the limited number of plants available for essential oils as well as the areas available for growing.

In a few areas with low pollution, people are farming plants whose essential oils are offered as derived "from organically grown plants." This means that no chemical fertilizers or pesticides have been used. These are the most valuable essences.

Looking at the overall environmental situation, we should be thankful that we can still purchase pure, natural essential oils. We should consider essential oils as jewels that can help us deal with our world and our bodies in a more careful and loving manner.

The Most Important Essential Oils

The following is an alphabetical list of the most important essential oils.

Basil	Fennel
Bergamot	Geranium
Camphor	Hyssop
Cedar	Jasmine
Chamomile	Juniper
Clary Sage	Lavender
Cypress	Lemon
Eucalyptus	Marjoram

Melissa   Rose
Myrrh   Rosemary
Neroli   Sandalwood
Orange   Sage
Patchouli   Tea Tree
Pepper   Thyme
Peppermint

4
Aromatherapy in Everyday Life

General Uses for the Body

We all have the option to take a drug (medicine) or visit a doctor when we experience such common distresses as headaches, digestion problems, stress, nervousness, loss of appetite, or insomnia. Or we can choose to help ourselves by using what nature has provided us in the form of essential oils and aromatherapy.

Aromatherapy is not intended to replace a visit to the doctor when we are troubled by a serious disease or permanent discomfort, but it can help us with many of our everyday ills. We can strengthen our immune system; influence the function of organs, glands, and hormones; fight bacteria, viruses, and fungi; sedate our nerves; tone and relax our muscles; and clear our minds.

Depending on the healing properties of the specific essential oil, we can treat ourselves for almost any disease and discomfort. This enables us to avoid drugs that can cause side effects and that have no life force. Essential oils help us in a natural manner without the danger of dependency, which drugs can create. You can use natural remedies by yourself or with the guidance of an aromatherapist. Healing and treating yourself includes taking responsibility for your health by looking for the causes of your discomfort, listening to your body's language, and becoming in tune with yourself.

Balancing Your Emotions

You can influence your emotions with scents. There are sedative scents, euphoric scents, aphrodisiac scents, and so forth. When inhaled, they will change your emotions significantly. The appropriate essential oil can provide relief from sadness, sorrow, anxiety, fear, depression, mood swings, anger, lethargy, and emotional numbness.

Aromatherapy helps balance your emotions, which in turn helps eradicate the causes of pain, tension, and diseases. These symptoms are often signals from your body that you have repressed emotions, or that something is going wrong in your life.

Sexuality

Sexuality is an important part of life. Sex brings us closer to another human being. This meeting charges our energy system and—if our partner is an appropriate one—makes us joyful and happy. Happiness is the root of a healthy and fulfilled life.

Essential oils can affect sexuality on three levels: First, they can directly trigger sexuality (by stimulating sexual hormones), and they relax the mind and body (by stimulating neurochemicals), which is a necessary step toward fulfilling sexuality. Second, they can also help to overcome impotence or anorgasmia with physical causes (by stimulating and strengthening the genitals and the reproductive system). And last but not least, a pleasant scent opens your heart to your partner.

See Chapter 9 for more on sexuality and essential oils.

Cosmetic Use

Our skin is the largest organ in the body. It comprises about five square feet of our body. It is exposed to a multitude of stressful elements, such as wind, cold, sun, polluted air, hard water, and poor nutrition. It is also an important organ for the excretion of toxins and wastes of the body.

Essential oils are used for a wide range of skin care. They are effective for treating burns, pimples, infections, fungi, inflammations, and irritations. Loss of hair, loss of hair color, and dandruff can also be successfully treated with essential oils.

Unlike pharmaceutical cosmetics, essential oils are, as stated earlier, a remedy with life force. How can a living cell be treated effectively with a dead substance? Many cosmetics contain animal substances. How can you treat your skin with substances having the vibrations of death and expect a healing or beneficial effect on a living body? Billions of animals die in the testing and production of cosmetics to satisfy the needs of the beauty industries. Essential oils offer a more humane *and* a more effective alternative.

Perfume

To deodorize, cover up, or change your body smell, you can use deodorants or perfumes. You may use perfumes for a variety of reasons: Maybe you don't like your smell, want to smell better, or want to be more attractive or lovable. Or you may use perfumes simply for your personal pleasure.

Perfume has been used throughout the centuries. In former times, it was the exclusive privilege of the upper classes. Until fairly recently, perfume was made only from natural ingredients, the scent being obtained from essential oils. Nowadays, commercial perfumes and most commercial cosmetics contain synthetic or "nature-identical" substances. Nature-identical substances are not natural. You, however, can use natural substances to create your own perfume with your own preferred scents. Essential oils, blended with a vegetable oil as a carrier, can please you and others as you learn more about the effects of particular scents. See Chapter 8 on how to create your own perfume.

Treatment of the Energy Centers

When either massaged on the energy centers (chakras) or inhaled, specific essential oils have beneficial effects. The field of influencing the chakras with essential oils is a relatively new one, but there are already a number of aromatherapists and energy therapists using scent to harmonize, open, and clear the energy centers. From my own experience, I can say that scent directly affects my chakras on all levels of being. See Chapter 12 for more on essential oils and the chakras.

Meditation and Spirituality

Knowledge of the effects of scents on your psyche enables you to use essential oils to relax, to meditate, to become centered, or to experience another level of being. Several essential oils have been used for centuries by various sects and religious groups to treat body *and* soul. Chapter 12 discusses spirituality and essential oils.

Cooking

Yes, you can use essential oils in the kitchen when preparing foods and drinks. You can use the concentrated form of herbs, fruit, roots, or spices in essential oils to give aroma to many things. With just a drop, you can turn your meal into a gourmet's delight. Remember to use only pure, natural oils. See Chapter 14 for more on cooking with essential oils.

Surrounding Yourself with Aroma

Natural scents can stimulate you with every breath you take. Essential oils can be used to create a pleasant smell in the rooms where you live or work, on your clothing, or in the bedding on which you sleep. Pleasing scents make you feel more comfortable. Essential oils can be used to scent nearly everything in your home; they refresh the air as well as fight the air's pathogens. They are also effective against insects. Instead of using artificial aromatics in washing powder and dish soap, you can use disinfecting, pleasant-smelling essential oils.

In the following chapters, we will explore the methods and recipes pertinent to the range of applications mentioned in this chapter.

5
Practical Applications of Essential Oils

The Aroma Lamp

With an aroma lamp or evaporator, you can give the air a particular aroma wherever you are. Simply by breathing, you can receive stimulating, healing effects without interrupting your activities. The aroma lamp is very helpful for infections of the respiratory system such as colds, flus, bronchitis, coughs, and asthma; it is also useful for overexcitement, nervousness, fatigue, insomnia, and exhaustion. Or you can simply use it to have a pleasant smell in your home, especially in winter.

Strong cooking odors can be eliminated by using certain essential oils in the aroma lamp. Insects avoid areas with certain scents, and bacterias and viruses in the air are successfully destroyed, or their growth inhibited, with particular scents. Aroma lamps can be very effective if you live with a sick person, because certain scents can prevent the spread of disease. By using the aroma lamp in your bedroom, you can treat yourself at night while sleeping. And in the office or workplace, scents can create an atmosphere conducive to creativity and concentration.

Modern aroma lamps are practical and usually well designed. You can choose between lamps with a small candle or electric ones with a bulb. The latter are more expensive but easier to handle as you do not have to replace the candle, which generally burns for about three hours. On top of any aroma lamp is a container to fill with water and the essential oil. Rinsing the container after each use prevents a blending of scents. The liquid in the container is supposed to evaporate slowly and should never boil or get very hot. This will destroy the beneficial properties of the oil. You should remember not to use the aroma lamp all day and not to change the scents within too short a period. If the liquid is completely evaporated, be sure to turn the lamp off. If you use an essential oil with a high scent intensity, you will still smell the scent even after many hours.

An electric diffuser (offered by several companies), or a bowl with water on a furnace, wood stove, or range, can be used as an alternative or to save electricity.

The average amount of oil to use in an aroma lamp is six to fifteen drops. But pay close attention to the odor intensity, as some oils have a very high intensity, in which case you'll need only two to three drops. You'll soon find the appropriate amount, as well as the appropriate aromas for your purpose, once you start your journey through the world of scents.

If you are a beginner at aromatherapy, test the scents in shops and start with those you find the most pleasing. Next, try some of the following recipes. The amount stated in the recipe refers to the number of drops of each essential oil for one blend.

Recipes for Use With Aroma Lamp

Refreshing and Disinfecting the Air
6 drops lavender or bergamot,
1 eucalyptus, 1 juniper

Strong Disinfectant, Antiseptic
4 drops hyssop, 4 cinnamon, 4 bergamot

Eliminating Cooking Odors
6 drops lemon, 6 orange

Headaches
4 drops Melissa, 2 peppermint
or Roman chamomile

Colds, Bronchitis
2 drops peppermint, 2 eucalyptus,
2 rosemary, 2 neroli

Heavy Cough, Asthma
6 drops hyssop
or
4 drops hyssop, 4 peppermint
or
2 drops eucalyptus, 2 benzoin, 2 thyme

Lack of Concentration, Mental Fatigue
2 drops lemongrass or Melissa,
2 peppermint, 2 basil
or
2 drops lemon, 1 bergamot, 4 peppermint

Peaceful and Relaxed Sleep
5 drops cedarwood, 1 lavender
or
3 drops rose
or
4 drops lavender, 2 neroli or bergamot

Insomnia
4 drops Roman chamomile, 2 lavender
or
4 drops neroli, 2 geranium
or
6 drops marjoram, 2 rosewood
or
6 drops lavender

The Aromatic Bath

Hearing the sound of running water, swimming in the ocean, and looking at a beautiful lake are relaxing experiences for most of us. Body and soul become peaceful. Human beings are almost always attached to water. Thousands of years ago, people all over the world built bathhouses, and bathing is still an important ritual of purification in many religions. Water cleanses the body and soul; it heals, relaxes, and rejuvenates.

If you live in a city, you may not find many opportunities to swim in a lake, sit peacefully by a creek, or take a swim in the ocean. But bathing in essential oils in your bathtub at home offers a variety of benefits. It can relax or stimulate body and mind, soothe or stimulate emotions, heal the body, aid in skin care, and, at the very least, provide a delightful scent experience. Bathing with essential oils is a very effective method of aromatherapy, as it combines the effects of both the essential oil and the water.

While taking a bath, you are stimulated by essential oils through the skin and the olfactory system. You smell the scent as the oil penetrates the skin. With warm water, the oil penetrates the skin quickly. Once the oils have penetrated the skin, body fluids such as the lymphs and the blood carry the oils through the body until the healing substances of the oil meet the appropriate systems, organs, cells, glands, and nerves. In addition, the skin is toned, deodorized, smoothed, rejuvenated, detoxified, and healed by the oil.

The recommended time for an aromatic bath is at least twenty minutes, which is as much time as the oil needs to penetrate the skin. Don't expect a sudden change in an illness or disease from bathing with essential oils. Oils are a subtle energy, and they require varying times depending on the condition of the skin (congested or uncongested) and the metabolism (slow or fast). However, stimulation of the emotions occurs quickly simply by breathing the scents in the bath. And the process of relaxation in a scented bath is important in this era of speed and stress.

Hints for an Aromatic Bath

In general, six to fifteen drops of essential oils are enough for a full bathtub. The hotter the water, the faster the oils dissolve and the faster they affect us. Since essential oils cannot dissolve by themselves in water, they should be blended with a vegetable oil, honey, or cream (milk). A bath with honey and cream makes the skin silky and nourishes the skin. Soap also dissolves the oils but also slows down their effects.

To begin your aromatic bath, fill the bathtub with water and get in. Wait a few minutes and then pour the essential oils into the water; by then, your skin is more receptive. To blend the water and the essential oil, move the water gently with your hand. You should never put the oil in an empty tub or under the running water, because it will evaporate before you enter the tub.

To dilute the oil and/or emulsify, you can use

- vegetable oil (two to three tablespoons)—this acts as a moisturizer and prevents your skin from dehydrating;
- honey (one tablespoon), or cream (whipped cream)—both act as emulsifying agents and both are beneficial for your skin;
- vinegar (two to three tablespoons)—this acts as an emulsifying agent and is helpful with blemished skin and oily skin;
- liquid soap, to prevent oily skin and to emulsify.

Recommended vegetable oils include jojoba oil, avocado oil, hazelnut oil, and almond oil. Almond oil activates the penetration of essential oils. Jojoba is not actually an oil but a wax that is useful for oily skin, acne, and inflamed skin. Using a blend of essential oils and vegetable oil, you will have an oily film on your skin after the bath, comparable to a body lotion. Don't rub this film off with a towel, as it contains essential oils. Give yourself time, wear a bathrobe, and let the lotion soothe and nourish your skin.

A final note: You can transform every ordinary bath time into a unique relaxing ceremony by putting on your favorite music and placing some candles in the bathroom. Engage all your senses in this special experience.

The following recipes are for full baths, hip baths, and foot baths. Again, the amounts in the recipes refer to *drops* of essential oils.

Recipes for Aromatic Baths

Full Baths

Stimulating and Refreshing Morning Bath
4 drops rosemary, 2 petitgrain
or
3 drops rosemary, 3 bergamot

Cleansing and Refreshing Bath
3 drops lemon, 3 geranium,
juice of one lemon (optional)
or
4 drops juniper, 2 rosemary, 2 fennel
or
3 drops thyme, 2 rosemary,
1 lavender, 1 peppermint

Relaxing Muscles
4 drops rosemary, 2 marjoram,
3 lavender or Roman chamomile

Colds, Flu, and Other Infections
3 drops lavender, 2 rosemary, 2 thyme
(stimulating; use in morning)
or
4 drops rosemary, 2 verbena

Depression, Fear
4 drops clary sage, 2 bergamot
or
6 drops Melissa, 4 basil

Nervousness, Overexcitement
6 drops geranium, 4 basil
or
4 drops lavender, 4 clary sage
or
5 drops orange, 1 jasmine

Mental Confusion
6 drops Melissa, 4 bergamot
or
6 drops lemon, 2 lemongrass, 2 lavender
or
4 drops rosewood, 4 patchouli

Shock
4 drops clary sage, 2 marjoram,
2 rose, 2 ylang-ylang
or
4 drops cypress, 2 cedarwood, 2 sandalwood

Relaxation, Meditation, Inner Silence
6 drops frankincense, 4 patchouli, 2 bergamot
3 drops lavender, 3 bergamot
(relaxing; use at night)

Nervousness, Excitement
4 drops geranium, 3 neroli or basil

Depression, Fear
4 drops lavender, 2 jasmine, 4 ylang-ylang

Shock
4 drops cypress, 4 cedarwood, 4 sandalwood

High Blood Pressure
4 drops ylang-ylang, 4 marjoram

Rheumatism
6 drops rosemary, 3 eucalyptus, 1 camphor

Detoxifying
2 drops geranium, 2 rosemary, 2 juniper

Cellulite
6 drops juniper, 2 orange, 2 cypress, 2 lemon
(two times a week, repeated for several months)

Fever
4 drops peppermint, 2 eucalyptus, 1 black pepper
(bathe only ten minutes, then go straight to bed)

Cramps, Colics
4 drops clary sage, 4 Roman chamomile

General Relaxation, Insomnia
4 drops Roman chamomile, 2 lavender
or
4 drops neroli, 2 Roman chamomile
or
3 drops lavender, 3 clary sage

or

4 drops lavender, 2 marjoram

Stimulating
6 drops rosemary, 2 bergamot

Toning muscles, Stimulating
3 drops rosemary, 2 juniper, 1 pepper

Hip Baths
(water only up to hips)

Hemorrhoids
5 drops cypress, 3 juniper, 3 frankincense

Impotence, Anorgasmia
6 drops clary sage, 2 jasmine, 2 pepper

Herpes on Sexual Organs
4 drops Melissa, 4 rose
or
6 drops bergamot

Infected Male Sexual Organs
4 drops sandalwood, 2 lavender, 1 rose

The following treatments can be made more effective with a vaginal douche or tampon. For a vaginal douche, the essential oils mentioned in the recipes should be stirred with one pint of warm water and flushed through the vagina using a douche bag. To use the recipes with a tampon, essential oils should be blended with one ounce of jojoba oil or almond oil; part of the blend should then be put on a tampon or natural sponge. Repeat each procedure several times a day. For more recipes for women, see Chapter 10.

Menstrual Cramps and Pain
4 drops clary sage, 3 marjoram, 2 peppermint
or
6 drops cypress, 2 clary sage

Irregular or Scanty Menstruation
4 drops clary sage, 3 Melissa, 1 rose

Vaginal Pruritus, Leukorrhea, Bacterias, and Fungus
3 drops Roman chamomile,
2 bergamot, 1 peppermint
or
2 drops rose, 4 lavender, 2 bergamot
or
4 drops lavender, 1 rose, 1 cinnamon
(especially if itching)
or
6 drops tea tree

Foot Baths

Foot baths give good results in treating headaches, migraines, menstrual cramps, colds, and tired, aching feet. The discipline of reflexology states that you can treat any organ through the reflex zones in the feet. You can use any of the blends mentioned in the recipes for full baths as foot baths. Getting a foot massage along with the foot bath is very beneficial. Here are additional recipes for foot baths:

Athlete's foot
6 drops tea tree or garlic
or
3 drops eucalyptus, 3 lavender

Perspiring Feet
3 drops cypress, 3 lavender, 3 sage
or
6 drops fir

Tired, Aching Feet
5 drops juniper, 2 rosemary

Internal Cramps and Aches
4 drops clary sage, 2 peppermint

Skin Irritants

Some essential oils can irritate the skin. The following oils should be used carefully. I recommend checking each of these oils for individual sensitivity; in particular, eucalyptus and camphor are very irritating to the skin. Use these oils sparingly.

Cajeput	Melissa
Camphor	Oregano
Cardamom	Pepper
Cedarwood	Peppermint
Citronella	Pennyroyal
Clove	Pine
Eucalyptus	Rosemary
Ginger	Sassafras
Lemon	Thyme
Lemongrass	

Massage

A good massage brings deep relaxation, and this effect can be greatly enhanced with essential oils. We all need to be touched and to feel close to other human beings; scented massage oils can bring an additional dimension to any method of massage.

There are two basic methods of aromatic massage in aromatherapy. The first is a full body massage, and the second is the massage of a certain area in order to treat a particular organ, muscles, or nerves.

The essential oil's penetration and effect on the body is similar to what happens in an aromatic bath. Here, the stimulation also works on two levels. Essences penetrate the skin and affect the organs, while the scent affects the olfactory sense and emotions.

As you are receiving a massage, or as you are giving yourself one, the essential oils slowly penetrate the skin, layer by layer. By using a dilution with vegetable oil, the skin is softened. The circulation and reproduction of new cells and the process of elimination of wastes are all intensified as your skin becomes more alive. After passing the first layer of skin, the essences enter the lymph and blood system, which carry them throughout the whole body. The process of penetration takes about twenty minutes. You should rest after the massage and enjoy the scent that surrounds you.

To dilute the essences, use vegetable oils. The best are cold-pressed, pure oils. Almond oil enhances the penetration of essences and is highly recommended for skin care because of its components. You can use any of the following oils:

Almond oil	Jojoba oil
Avocado oil	Sunflower oil
Hazelnut oil	Wheat germ oil

As previously mentioned, jojoba is a liquid wax of the jojoba plant. It makes the skin silky and soft. You can prevent oxidation of your massage oil by adding ten percent wheat germ oil to any blend (except for jojoba oil, which never turns rancid).

When mixing a blend for a massage oil, you will want to prepare a larger quantity than for just one massage. The average quantities for blends are:

- ten to twenty drops of essential oils for a one percent dilution with two ounces of carrier oil (for balancing emotions, mind, and nerves); or
- up to sixty drops for a three percent dilution with two ounces of carrier oil (for the healing of internal ailments).

The effects of scents on the emotions and spirit are more intense if the massage oil contains a small quantity of essential oils. It is the fine fragrance that stimulates, not the amount of scent.

Recipes for Aromatic Massage

The following quantities are based on using two ounces of vegetable oil.

Stimulating
15 drops rosewood, 6 geranium, 4 orange

Relaxing
15 drops lavender, 10 sandalwood, 5 Melissa

Strengthening the Immune System
20 drops lavender, 5 bergamot

Aching Muscles
10 drops juniper, 8 rosemary,
8 lavender, 2 lemon

Weakness of Connective Tissue
30 drops lavender, 50 ml. wheat germ oil

Tired, Aching Legs
15 drops rosemary, 10 lavender

Cellulite
15 drops orange, 10 cypress
or
10 drops cypress, 6 geranium, 3 sage
(with wheat germ and jojoba oil)

Varicose Veins
10 drops juniper, 10 cypress, 5 lemon
or
10 drops rosemary, 6 juniper, 6 lavender
(use daily, but do not massage the veins directly)

Smoothing the Skin
15 drops lavender, 4 neroli, 4 rose or frankincense

Reducing Weight, Draining the Tissue, Increasing Circulation
(especially in the hips and thighs)
20 drops juniper, 10 cypress

Bust Growth
15 drops ylang-ylang, 10 geranium

Rheumatism
10 drops juniper, 10 rosemary,
5 lavender, 5 lemon
or
10 drops camphor, 15 rosemary, 10 eucalyptus
(test skin sensitivity first)

Sedative for Sorrow, Depression, Overexcitement
8 drops bergamot, 8 rosewood, 2 jasmine
or
8 drops ylang-ylang, 4 patchouli or jasmine

Headaches or Cold and Flu Aches
2 drops Melissa or lavender undiluted
on forehead and/or temples

Mental Exhaustion
2 drops Melissa undiluted on forehead
and temples

Dizziness, Lack of Memory
2 drops rosemary undiluted on
forehead and temples

If you are working in the field of massage, body work, or therapy, you will need large quantities of massage oil. Just multiply the amounts of drops of essential oil and carrier oil to manufacture your stock of massage oils. Always store the massage oils in amber-colored (dark) glass bottles and add wheat germ oil so they won't turn rancid. Of course, you can also give any moisturizer or ready-made massage oil a specific scent by stirring in essential oils. Please note: It is important to let your new blends settle a few days so carrier oil and essential oil can merge.

Inhalation

Inhalation is especially beneficial for infections of the respiratory system and sinuses, congestion of the sinuses, colds, flus, asthma, coughs, headaches, and migraines. When you breathe in the essential oils, they are carried immediately to the site of disease, and the effects are instantaneous. Since inhalation affects the entire body as well as the mind and emotions, you can use inhalation for any desired healing process; however, inhalation is usually used for the discomforts just mentioned.

When essential oils are inhaled, they can prevent the growth of viruses, eliminate bacteria, relax aches, and act as sedatives or expectorants.

In preparing inhalants, combine no more than two pints of hot water with a maximum of six drops of essential oil (use only two to three drops for thyme and sage) in a bowl and completely cover your head and the bowl with a large towel. Be careful that the water's steam is not too hot, and inhale through your nose. Do this for at least ten minutes. This method also serves as a superb facial steam.

You can also try dry inhalation. This means you simply put two to three drops of essential oils on a tissue and inhale. Wherever you are, in a train, in a car, on a plane, or at work, you can use this simple method. This method helps you avoid catching infectious diseases, which are easily spread in closed rooms and on public transportation. For those of you who suffer in airplanes from headaches, dry noses, or the fear of flying, use the simple blend of one drop bergamot, one lavender, and one peppermint on a tissue.

For nasal congestion, create an effective nose spray that won't dry out your nose with ten ml. hazelnut oil, and add four drops of the appropriate essential oils as mentioned in the following recipes for inhalations.

Recipes for Inhalation

The following recipes are based on using two pints of hot water.

Headache
1 drop Melissa, 2 peppermint, 2 lavender

Colds or Flu
2 drops eucalyptus, 2 peppermint, 2 tea tree
or
1 drop sage, 2 lemongrass, 4 rosemary

Strong Flu
4 drops eucalyptus, 1 camphor, 1 pepper

Throat Infection
3 drops thyme

Aiding in Removal of Mucus
from Respiratory System
Choose from hyssop, bergamot, sandalwood,

eucalyptus, basil, marjoram, peppermint.
(Use a total of 6 drops.)

Congested or Infected Sinuses (Sinusitis)
Choose from eucalyptus, basil,
peppermint, thyme, tea tree.
(Use a total of 6 drops.)

Asthma
3 drops hyssop, 2 lavender, 1 peppermint

Deepening the Breathing
4 drops frankincense

Compresses

Hot or cold compresses are an ancient method of healing aches, cramps, colics, swellings, wrenched tendons and muscles, sprains, falls, and bruises. The essential oils are concentrated on the appropriate area and thereby take effect quickly and specifically. Water, itself a healer, helps the oils to penetrate the skin. Leave the compress on for at least twenty minutes.

Hot compresses are useful for rheumatism, arthritis, neuralgia, aching muscles, back pain, cramps, menstrual pain, toothaches, earaches, colics, fever, bronchitis, skin inflammation, and abscesses. Hot compresses are also widely applied for cosmetic purposes. You can treat the facial skin very successfully with compresses as you will see in the recipes.

Cold compresses are useful for headaches, swellings, wrenched tendons and pulled muscles, bruises, sprains, falls, tennis elbow, and eye aches or tension.

Compresses should be changed as soon as they reach the body's temperature. Hot compresses can be covered with a dry towel to keep in the heat.

Special note: *Never make compresses for the eyes with an undiluted oil.* Compresses for the eyes must be highly diluted.

Recipes for Aromatic Compresses

A basic dilution for compresses is five to ten drops of essential oil in two pints of water. Stir the dilution thoroughly, then soak a towel in the water, wring it to remove the excess water, put the compress on the area, and rest. Change compresses as soon as they reach the body's temperature.

Hot Compresses

Aching Muscles
2 drops Roman chamomile, 2 rosemary, 1 sandalwood

Colics
2 drops basil, 2 rosemary, 1 fennel

Cramps (Menstruation)
3 drops clary sage, 2 marjoram

Basic Pain-Relieving Blend
2 drops peppermint, 2 lavender, 2 Roman chamomile
(For more pain-relieving oils, see Chapter 18.)

Acne, Pimples
2 drops lavender, 1 lemon

Dry Skin
2 drops rose, 1 neroli, 1 Roman chamomile

Oily Skin
1 drop rose, 1 sandalwood, 1 geranium

Irritated Skin
2 drops blue chamomile, 1 rose

Inflamed, Sensitive Skin
2 drops blue chamomile, 1 rose

Rejuvenating the Skin
2 drops vetiver, 1 neroli

Cold Compresses

Headache or Sunstroke
3 drops rose, 1 Melissa, 1 lavender

Fever
2 drops lemon, 1 lavender
(on forehead)
or
2 drops eucalyptus
(on feet)

Nervousness and Stress
4 drops lavender, 1 Melissa
(on forehead)

Sprains, Falls, and Bruises
2 drops lavender, 2 fennel

Headache or Hangover
4 drops geranium, 1 lemon

Compresses for Eyes

Dilute the essential oil with one cup of water and apply with a cotton pad. Leave the soaked cotton pad on your closed eyes for at least ten minutes. Remember that compresses for the eyes must always be highly diluted.

Inflamed, Tired Eyes or Conjunctivitis
1 drop rose or Roman chamomile or lavender

Internal Use

The internal use of essential oils is a common treatment in some countries (such as France, England, Italy, and Germany), whereas in other countries this application is not recommended or allowed, or has not been approved by national control organizations, such as in the United States. You should only take essential oils for internal use if you are under the supervision of an aromatherapist who is also a physician.

Remember that essential oils are highly concentrated. The layperson does not always know which substances are in a particular oil. Administering essences internally can be dangerous or cause unpleasant side effects. Absolute oils such as rose, tuberose, violet, or jasmine, for example, contain chemical solubles and are not recommended for internal use at all.

In any case, essential oils have a very strong taste, and many people cannot swallow them. They may even make some people vomit.

Unsupervised internal use of essential oils can do more harm than good. You should *never* attempt a long-term cure by yourself, and *never* give essential oils to children internally.

I have personally taken essential oils internally, and I have often experienced an overreaction in both my stomach and colon. Perhaps the problem was due to the oil not being pure, original, and genuine, or perhaps I took too strong a dose. Many people assume that a larger quantity of oil will cure them faster and better, but that's not the case. Even the smallest amounts can have strong effects on your body's systems.

So far in this book, I have stressed practical and safe applications that can enable you to be a "self-healer." I recommend sticking with these particular applications.

I will, however, mention a few recipes here that are useful for a variety of discomforts and that are also safe. When using essential oils for internal use, remember to use only pure, genuine oils.

Recipes for Internal Use

Take the following recipes with a big glass of warm water and honey, stirring the contents vigorously. Drink the blend slowly, taking fifteen minutes between sips. Or drop the oils into a gelatin capsule. This prevents you from tasting the sometimes unpleasant, strong taste. For treating stomach discomfort, be certain to *taste* the essential oil, as the taste buds ignite the curative process. You should never use more than three drops three times a day.

Vomiting, Nausea, and Mild Digestive Problems
3 drops peppermint or basil

Heartburn
2 drops sandalwood

Constipation, Stomach Cramps, and Nausea, or as Digestive Aid
1 drop basil, 1 Roman chamomile, 1 peppermint,
1 juniper or fennel

Headaches
2 drops peppermint

Cramps
3 drops clary sage

Coughs
1 drop hyssop

Whooping Coughs
2 drops hyssop, 2 cypress

Nervousness of Stomach and Colon
2 drops geranium

Hangovers
1 drop peppermint, 1 fennel

Gargles

Antiseptic Blend for Inflammation, Ulcers, or Sores of the Mouth and Throat
2 drops bergamot, 1 lavender, 1 peppermint
or
2 drops lemon, 2 peppermint
(in one glass of water, stirred well)

Sore Throat (Streptococcus or Staphylococcus)
3 drops sandalwood or onion
(in one glass of water, stirred vigorously;
gargle only—do not drink)

Mouthwashes
Mouthwashes with essential oils can be very helpful for bad breath, oral infections, and gums. The following blends should be gargled but never swallowed.

Disinfectant Mouthwash
3 drops bergamot, 2 lavender
(in 1 glass of water, stirred well)

Bad Breath
2 drops bergamot, 1 peppermint
(in 1 glass of water, stirred well)

Mouthwash
3 drops peppermint, 3 thyme, 1 fennel
(to make a large amount, mix in 16 ounces of
distilled water, with 2 tablespoons of vodka
or brandy)

Fresh Breath and Healthy Gums
1 drop peppermint, 1 thyme, 1 myrrh
(in ½ pint of water, stirred vigorously)

6
Specific Treatments

Recipes for Treating Common Physical Ailments

Abscesses, Cold
Apply hot compress with bergamot, lavender, Roman chamomile, garlic, or tea tree.

Abscesses, Warm
Apply cold compress with onion.

Athlete's Foot
Take a morning and evening foot bath with tea tree or myrrh and lavender. Or use body oil of 2 oz. carrier oil, 15 drops lavender, 15 myrrh, or 40 drops tea tree.

Bleeding
Apply one of the following oils diluted with some water dabbed with cotton on the wound: eucalyptus, geranium, lemon, rose, or pennyroyal.

Bronchitis
(1) Inhale rosemary for five minutes several times a day.

(2) Rub chest several times a day with a blend of 2 oz. carrier oil, 80 drops thyme, and 20 lavender.
(3) Apply a chest wrap with 2 pints hot water, 10 drops thyme, 2 lavender.

Bruises
Apply a cold compress with fennel, camphor, lavender, and/or hyssop.

Burns
Dab or lay a cloth with lavender on the spot. Aloe vera mixed with lavender is also helpful.

Cellulite
(1) Massage daily with a blend of 2 oz. wheat germ oil, 20 drops oregano, 10 geranium.
(2) Bathe in a hip bath two times a week for several months with 6 drops juniper, 2 orange, 2 cypress.

Cuts
Apply an ointment of lavender, bergamot, and eucalyptus. (See the recipe in Chapter 7.)

Eczemas
Rub daily with 2 oz. aloe vera, 15 drops lavender, 15 immortelle.

Fungal Skin Infection
Rub daily with a blend of 2 oz. jojoba oil, 20 drops tea tree, 10 lavender.

Fungal Toenail Infection
Brush the lower side of the nails with a blend of alcohol, lavender, and myrrh once a day for one week. After this, continue with the athlete's foot treatment.

Inflammation of the Middle Ear
Blend 20 eucalyptus, 5 lavender. Shake vigorously. Drip two drops of the blend on a cotton and place in the ear. Or put the drops in the ear with your finger. Rub the surrounding area with diluted lavender.

Mouth Ulcer
Dab 2 drops myrrh on the ulcer.

Nose Bleeds
Put 2 drops lemon in icy water and saturate a cotton pad with the mixture. Place cotton pad in the nose.

Sore Skin
Rub with a blend of 1 oz. almond oil, 4 drops rose.

Sunburn
Bathe with 6 drops peppermint, 4 lavender.

Tonsillitis
Gargle several times daily with a blend of 20 drops bergamot, 20 thyme, 5 cinnamon. Use two drops of this blend in a glass of water to gargle.

Varicose Veins
Every day, rub the area surrounding the veins with a blend of 4 oz. almond oil, 20 drops rosemary, 20 juniper, 10 lemon.

Warts

Dab undiluted camphor, lavender, or eucalyptus on warts daily (do not use on genital warts).

Wounds and Inflammation

The following oils are generally helpful: benzoin, bergamot, blue chamomile, eucalyptus, geranium, immortelle, lavender, myrrh, peppermint, and tea tree.

7
Skin and Hair Care

As mentioned earlier, the skin is the largest organ of the human body and, along with the heart and the liver, one of the most important ones.

The skin's tasks are various. It covers and protects your body, breathes, eliminates poisons and wastes, manufactures vitamins, adjusts the body's temperature, excretes liquids, grows hair, absorbs harmful and beneficial substances, warns of burns and hurts, and gives the senses information on hot, warm, cold, wet, dry, soft, rough, pleasant, and so forth.

The skin reflects on the outside how the body functions on the inside; as the old saying goes, "As without, so within." The skin attempts to excrete all the poisons and toxins that the inner organs cannot eliminate, including those found in food, alcohol, nicotine, and caffeine. The skin reveals, through various symptoms, the lack of a balanced, healthy diet as well as a lack of liquid. Unfortunately, most people don't drink enough water or eat enough vitamin-rich food. Insufficient intake of liquids damages the function of the skin, and vitamin deficiency causes deterioration of the skin.

Many common physical conditions affect the skin. Extreme changes in the hormonal balance, occurring mostly in women during menstruation and menopause, result in irritated skin.

Our emotions also affect skin condition. Any extreme mood swings, or dramatic changes of life, can result in a worsening condition of the skin. The skin is a vent for many organic and emotional processes. It also has to deal with outside elements: wind, water, sun, dust, and toxins in the air. This is only a short, incomplete description of the tasks and functions of the skin. It is meant to convey how important the skin really is.

The skin is made up of three layers. The first layer is visible and is called the epidermis. It contains dead or dying cells. Cells from the lower layers move toward this uppermost layer in a continual process of elimination and renewal. This demonstrates the importance of thorough and appropriate cleansing of the skin. The faster the renewal, the smoother the skin looks. If the lifeless cells cling too long to the skin, it will look dead, dry, and old.

The second layer of the skin is called the dermis. It contains sweat glands, sebaceous glands, blood vessels, sensory nerves, and hair follicles.

The third layer of the skin is called the subcutaneous. This bottom layer contains muscles and fat tissue. If the functions of this thin layer of skin are impaired, if its channels are clogged and liquids are unable to travel, you will not have healthy skin or a healthy appearance.

Aromatherapy can help to correct imbalances of the skin. The essential oils contain various substances that cleanse, disinfect, stimulate, hydrate, rejuvenate, smoothe, heal, sedate, and nourish the three layers of the skin.

Hair is comprised of dead cells, but hair growth depends on healthy skin. Therefore, essential oils are also helpful for hair care. Softness, color, shine, and a full head of hair are all enhanced with essential oils.

Although commercial cosmetics may offer the same results, they contain mostly synthetic substances that only improve the skin's condition for a short period at best. And they are overpriced when compared to their ingredients. These cosmetics work mostly at the surface and may actually damage sensitive skin.

Many commercial products use animal substances, and, as I've already stated, how can substances from slaughtered animals, which carry the vibrations of death, improve or heal living cells? Do we really want animals to die to provide us with eternal youth and beauty? The producers of some natural cosmetics do not use animal substances in their products and do not test their products on animals.

The science of natural healing and healing with herbs is as old as humanity and has been proven effective over the centuries; only harmless plants and essences are used in the production of natural cosmetics. With essential oils, you are maintaining and correcting your skin with living nature.

Basic Hints for Skin and Hair Care

With a few exceptions, such as the treatment of pimples, insect bites, warts, and burns, essential oils should not be applied undiluted to the skin. To dilute essences, use cold-pressed, pure vegetable oils (referred to as carrier oils), natural creams, natural shampoos, distilled, pure water, or springwater. The recommended carrier oils are almond oil, avocado oil, jojoba oil, olive oil, peanut oil, sunflower oil, and wheat germ oil. You can prevent the oxidation of a blend and provide the skin with vitamin E by adding ten percent wheat germ oil. I usually add one teaspoon of pure vitamin E oil to all facial oils. The blends will then last for one year if stored in a cool, dark place in airtight containers.

Blends of essential oils and carrier oils should be stirred or shaken vigorously. Then let them settle for a few days so the essential oils and the vegetable oil can merge with one another.

Facial oils should be left on your face for fifteen minutes before removing the excess oil. Masks can be prepared with yogurt, honey, avocado, wheat germ oil, lemon, and clay. All of these should be natural, of course. Leave the mask on the face for twenty minutes. Then rinse with warm water and dry the skin gently. Don't cover the skin afterward with makeup, as it is best to allow the skin to breathe.

Now let's take a look at the general uses of essential oils for the skin.

Treatment of the Face and the Body

Normal Skin
bergamot, cedarwood, geranium, lavender, neroli, Roman chamomile, rose, rosewood

Dry Skin
cedarwood, geranium, jasmine, lavender,
orange, rose, rosewood, ylang-ylang

Oily Skin
bergamot, camphor, cedarwood, cypress,
frankincense, geranium, juniper,
lavender, lemon, rose

Sensitive Skin
jasmine, orange, Roman chamomile, rose

Irritated Skin
blue chamomile, rose

Mature (Aging) Skin
cypress, fennel, frankincense, lavender, myrrh,
neroli, orange, patchouli, rose, vetiver

Inflamed Skin
blue chamomile, carrot seed, geranium,
hyssop, immortelle, myrrh, peppermint, rose,
sandalwood, tea tree

Acne
bergamot, cajeput, camphor, geranium,
immortelle, juniper, lavender, Roman chamomile,
rose, tea tree

Chapped Skin
benzoin, blue chamomile, carrot seed,
geranium, lavender, patchouli, rose, sandalwood

Rejuvenation and Cell Regeneration
all oils, especially frankincense, lavender,
neroli, rose, sandalwood, tea tree

Sebum Balance
bergamot

Sebum Reduction
juniper, lemon

Pimples
lavender, lemon, tea tree (undiluted)

Freckles
lemon, onion

Skin Cleansing
basil, juniper, lemon, niaouli, peppermint

Deodorants
benzoin, bergamot, clary sage,
cypress (for feet), eucalyptus, lavender,
neroli, patchouli, pine, rosewood

Dermatitis, Inflammations and Diseases of the Skin
blue chamomile, cajeput, carrot seed,
cinnamon, clove, eucalyptus, hyssop,
immortelle, juniper, myrrh, onion,
peppermint, sage, sandalwood, thyme

Cellulite
cypress, juniper, lavender,
orange, oregano, rosemary

Fungal Infections and Athlete's Foot
eucalyptus, garlic, lavender, tea tree

Itching Skin
cedarwood, jasmine, peppermint,
Roman chamomile

Hand Care (Chapped Skin)
lemon, myrrh, onion, rose, sandalwood

Treatment of the Nails

Brittle Nails
lemon, onion

Nail Care
cypress, lavender, sandalwood

Treatment of the Hair

Generally Effective on the Hair
cedarwood, clary sage, cypress, juniper,
lavender, lemon, Roman chamomile,
rosemary, rosewood, sage

Oily Hair
cedarwood, clary sage, cypress, juniper, lavender

Dandruff
eucalyptus, rosemary

Hair Loss
cedarwood, juniper, sage, tea tree

Recipes for Cosmetics

Numerous recipes exist for natural cosmetics.
Another book would be needed to describe all the

recipes and their effects. I will mention a few recipes for each problem, disorder, or symptom, thus enabling you to vary them with the selection of oils mentioned earlier in the chapter.

The amounts produced in the following recipes will be more than enough for one treatment. To produce an even greater supply, simply double or triple the amounts. All blends have to be shaken or stirred well. Remember to store them in a dark, cool place to guarantee a long-lasting blend.

Facial Oils

Facial oils nourish and stimulate the skin. They also protect it from the elements, and keep it from becoming too dry. Clean your hands before applying oils to the skin; otherwise, you might apply not only the oil but also bacteria and germs.

All recipes are based on a carrier of two ounces vegetable oil, such as jojoba, almond, or avocado oil. It is very nourishing to blend one-half ounce of wheat germ oil and one-half ounce of any other vegetable oil. For oily skin and acne, I especially recommend jojoba oil. Do not use a mineral oil.

Dry Skin
10 drops sandalwood, 7 geranium,
5 ylang-ylang, 3 rosewood

Oily Skin
15 drops lemon, 12 cypress or camphor,
10 lavender

Acne
15 drops bergamot, 10 juniper, 6 cypress
or
15 drops tea tree

Mature (Aging) Skin
15 drops lavender, 5 frankincense,
4 neroli, 4 rose

Inflamed or Irritated Skin
10 drops sandalwood, 5 blue chamomile, 5 rose
or
2 drops clove, 1 cinnamon, 3 blue chamomile

Wrinkles
15 drops fennel, 5 lavender, 5 rose

Normal Skin
15 drops lavender, 8 geranium, 4 rose

Facial Steaming

Steaming the face with essential oils hydrates the skin, cleanses the pores, and stimulates at the same time. After the steaming, you should treat the skin with a light facial cream, a facial oil, or toner. The recipes given here are based on using one to two pints of hot water.

Normal Skin
4 drops lavender, 4 geranium, 4 patchouli

Oily Skin and Acne
6 drops juniper, 4 lemon, 4 cypress

Facial Compresses

Compresses have a humidifying and stimulating effect similar to steaming, but the oil is absorbed by the skin more quickly with compresses. The skin becomes very smooth and soft, and breathing in the pleasant scents is a very stimulating experience in itself. The recipes given here are based on using one to two pints of hot water.

Acne
2 drops lavender, 2 juniper or 1 lemon,
1 bergamot
or
4 drops tea tree

Dry Skin
2 drops rose, 1 Roman chamomile, 1 neroli

Oily Skin
1 drop rose, 1 sandalwood, 1 geranium

Inflamed or Irritated Skin
2 drops blue chamomile, 1 myrrh,
2 hyssop or 1 rose

Mature (Aging) Skin
2 drops vetiver, 1 frankincense,
2 myrrh or 1 neroli

Facial Toner

Facial toners prepared with essential oils balance and stimulate the skin. Apply the toner after cleansing the skin. You might choose to use toners instead of facial oils, which can be too greasy for oily skin.

Dry or Normal Skin
4 drops lavender, 2 geranium
(in 2 oz. springwater or distilled water)
or
20 drops rose, 8 Roman chamomile
(in 8 oz. rose water mixed with ¼ oz.
alcohol, such as vodka)

Oily Skin
4 drops bergamot, 2 lavender
(in 2 oz. springwater or distilled water)
or
6 drops bergamot, 4 lavender
(in 8 oz. rose water mixed with ¼ oz.
alcohol, such as vodka)

All-Purpose Toner
8 drops geranium, 8 bergamot,
4 cypress, 2 lavender
(in 16 oz. springwater or distilled water)

Facial Masks

Facial masks prepared with essential oils stimulate and deeply cleanse the skin. Clay masks are the best, as clay acts as a magnet to toxins. It contains cleansing minerals such as silica, iron, magnesium, zinc, and calcium. To prepare the mask, use a bowl and stir all the ingredients of the mask until they are pastelike. Then spread the mask on your face. Leave clay masks on the skin for fifteen minutes and then rinse them off with warm water. Leave other masks on for five minutes. Keep the masks in airtight containers in a cool and dry place, preferably in the refrigerator.

Normal, Dry, and Sensitive Skin
1 drop lavender, 1 geranium
(Mix with 2 Tbsp. natural clay, 1 tsp.
avocado or honey, and 2 tsp. water.)

Acne
1 drop juniper, 1 bergamot
(Mix with 2 Tbsp. clay, 1 Tbsp. yogurt,
and 2 tsp. water.)

Mature (Aging) Skin
1 drop frankincense, 1 myrrh
(Mix with 2 Tbsp. clay, 1 Tbsp. honey
or avocado, and 2 tsps. water.)

Oily Skin
1 drop camphor, 1 juniper
(Mix with 2 Tbsp. clay, 1 Tbsp. lemon fruit,
and 2 tsps. water or honey.)

Body Lotions and Body Oils
The following recipes are based on using four
ounces of vegetable oil.

General Care
20 drops rose (10 percent diluted), 5 lavender
(Mix with 3 oz. almond oil and 1 oz. jojoba oil.)

Irritated Skin
7 drops Roman chamomile, 7 rose, 5 geranium
(in 4 oz. jojoba oil)

Mature (Aging) Skin
7 drops frankincense, 7 lavender, 5 patchouli
(Mix with 3 oz. almond oil and 1 oz. jojoba oil.)

Oily Skin
7 drops cedarwood, 7 cypress, 5 frankincense
(in 4 oz. jojoba oil)

Cellulite
10 drops juniper, 7 rosemary, 4 lavender
(in 4 oz. jojoba oil)

Weakened Connective Tissue
30 drops rosewood, 10 rose
(Mix with 4 oz. jojoba oil and 4 oz.
wheat germ oil.)

Creams

Creams sometimes clog the pores of the skin. The use of facial oils is almost always sufficient, but I want to mention at least one basic recipe to produce a cream.

Blend forty grams of oil, forty grams of water, ten grams of beeswax, and ten to fifteen drops of essential oils. Or blend fifty grams of oil, forty grams of cacao butter, ten grams of beeswax, forty grams of water, and twenty drops of essential oils. Heat the oils and the beeswax until the ingredients are melted. Then add the separately heated water very slowly, as in making a mayonnaise. Beat the mix constantly with a rotary whisk until all the water is absorbed. Make sure you stop as soon as all the water is absorbed. Finally, add the essential oils by stirring them in gently.

Use stainless steel bowls to prepare creams. Put the cream in little pots or jars, and keep them in the refrigerator. Keep only small containers in the bathroom. The creams will last for up to two months.

All-Purpose Cream
10 grams lanolin anhydrite, 5 grams beeswax,
5 grams cacao butter, 40 grams almond oil,
40 grams rose water,
10–20 drops of essential oils
(Melt the lanolin, wax, and cacao butter together until all the substances become liquid. Add almond oil and bring the heat up to 140 degrees. Remove the container from the heat and add the rose water by stirring continuously. Continue stirring with the mixer on the lowest speed until the paste becomes cold. Finally, add the essential oils while stirring a minute more.)

You may prefer to buy an unscented, natural cream, such as aloe vera cream, or vegetable jelly and add the preferred essential oils. This will save you the trouble of preparing your own cream from scratch.

Ointment for Wounds

To make an effective ointment for healing wounds, combine 2 ounces of vegetable jelly or rich natural cream, 10 drops bergamot or Roman chamomile, 10 lavender, and 5 eucalyptus. Stir in the essential oils and store the ointment in a jar in the refrigerator.

Hand Care

You can make a rich hand cream from 2 ounces of vegetable jelly or aloe vera cream. Add 5 drops myrrh, 5 rose, and 5 sandalwood.

Nail Care

Cracked nails can be treated with a blend of one-half ounce of vegetable oil and 20 drops of lemon. For a basic nail-care formula, blend one ounce of vegetable oil, 4 drops lavender, 4 cypress, and 4 sandalwood. Soak your fingernails for ten minutes in the blend, or dab it on the toenails.

Hair Care

For strong, healthy hair, it is very important to clean the hair, brush it thoroughly, massage the scalp, and use a shampoo containing keratin, a protein with eighteen amino acids that is a component of the hair and skin. The growth of the hair starts in the hair bulb underneath the skin. As you know by now, essential oils stimulate the skin and also encourage the growth of the hair. Mixed with shampoos, they enhance the cleansing process, soothe the scalp, and also refresh the hair's color. Use Roman chamomile and lemon for blond or light-colored hair, sandalwood and rosemary for dark hair. Sandalwood gives dark hair an especially nice shine.

Shampoo

To produce your own scented shampoo, buy a natural, nondetergent shampoo and enrich it with essential oils. A guide follows, based on using sixteen ounces of shampoo. Shake all blends well.

Dry Hair
10 drops cedarwood

Oily Hair
10 drops rosemary

Normal Hair
10 drops lavender or Roman chamomile

Hair Loss
3 drops cedarwood, 3 rosemary

Dandruff
5 drops rosemary, 5 cedarwood
or
10 drops rosemary

Hair Rinse

After cleansing with shampoo, use an aromatic water as a rinse. Take sixteen ounces of water and add five to ten drops of essential oil.

Light Hair
lemon, Roman chamomile

Dark Hair
rosemary, rosewood or sandalwood

Oily Hair or Dandruff
clary sage, lavender

Hair Cure

Once in a while, nourish your hair with a hair cure, especially if you have been exposed to too much sun or wind. You should also use a hair cure when you feel that your hair is becoming too thin or dry.

Even oily hair needs nutrition, although it sounds like a paradox to treat oily hair with an oil cure. But the essential oils treat the skin that is producing the oily hair. Leave the following cures on your hair for at least twenty minutes (and up to two hours) and later shampoo several times. The blends use a base of two to three ounces of olive oil, or, for even better results, use jojoba oil.

Oily Hair
10 drops cypress, 10 cedarwood, 8 juniper

Dandruff
10 drops eucalyptus, 20 rosemary
(Leave on for two hours.)

Normal Hair
10 drops lavender, 20 cedarwood or rosewood
(Leave on for twenty minutes.)

8
Creating Your Own Perfume

The word "perfume" comes from the French expression *per fume*—by burning or smoke. This expression has its roots in the old method of burning incense, which was practiced for centuries in Egypt and the Orient. Until the discovery of synthesizing, perfumes were comprised of essential oils and a fixative. Contemporary commercial perfumes are made mostly of synthetics and a few essential oils.

Perfume enhances our attractiveness to others. We balance or manipulate our body's smell with perfume and feel much better as a consequence of our pleasant scent.

The scents of essential oils vary from earthy to light, from sweet to woody, from flowery to musky. You can create your own perfume by choosing any one of these various characteristics. Unlike synthetic perfume, natural scents will cause more of a reaction in the brain, so you need to consider how the scents affect your moods as well as how others will react to you.

To create your own perfume, combine a carrier oil (such as jojoba oil) and the essential oils you select. It is best to begin with a simple blend of essential oils whose scent you find pleasant. Famous perfumes are sometimes made of up to two hundred different scents! You'll do better if you use only a few and wait for the results of your first homemade perfume. For a basic perfume, blend one-quarter of an ounce of jojoba oil with twenty-five to thirty drops of essential oil. Then keep the bottle closed for at least one week to allow the scents to merge.

The manufacturing is simple, but not the composing. Composing a perfume is like composing music. The scents are like the instruments of an orchestra, which must perform together to make music. The music of the perfume is the ultimate outcome.

As you experiment with making your own perfumes, you will learn to differentiate between "top scents" (which you smell at first and which evaporate quickly), "middle scents" (which provide the main character of the perfume and which are medium lasting), and "basic scents" (which you still smell at the end of evaporation and which last the longest). You must also remember to consider the intensity of the scents.

You can balance the intensity of the different scents by varying the amounts of essential oils. Make sure that one scent doesn't dominate or repress the other ones with its intensity. In the appendix at the end of the book, you will find a table listing the rates of intensity and evaporation for the most common essential oils.

Recipes for Some Basic Perfumes

The following recipes are based on using one-quarter ounce of jojoba oil.

Tangy, Masculine
15 drops sandalwood, 5 cedarwood,
5 rosewood, 2 lemongrass

Light, Sweet
4 drops rose, 4 rosewood,
2 neroli, 4 cedarwood

Very Sweet
8 drops rosewood, 4 jasmine,
4 ylang-ylang, 1 vanilla, 1 bergamot

Flowery
10 drops bergamot, 8 geranium,
5 neroli, 5 vetiver

Heavy, Musky
10 drops patchouli, 8 sandalwood,
4 ylang-ylang, 4 rose, 4 jasmine

9

The Sexual Response

In ancient Rome, rose petals were strewn on the marital bed to stimulate the couple's sexuality. Cleopatra is said to have bolstered her sensuality with the scent of jasmine. There is a long history of using scents as aphrodisiacs and, indeed, scents can enhance your sexuality. Scent information is transmitted directly to the limbic system of the brain, which is closely connected with the parts of your brain that influence sex and control hormones.

In the animal realm, smell is a determining factor for the selection of a mate and for sexual impulses. The olfactory systems of many animals are much more developed and enable them to find the right partner across long distances, even if the wind is carrying the scent molecules in another direction. Animals can differentiate among the scents in a herd of thousands of animals and can thus locate their partners and their offspring.

Humans have to come into closer contact in order to recognize one another's smells. Our sexuality is mostly triggered by the scent of sexual hormones. These are released by our sweat. But the connection between scent and sexuality can be a subtle one, and individual tastes vary. Whatever our preferences, though, the smell of our partner's body is important for attraction, sympathy, sensuousness, and love.

Many famous perfumes contain aphrodisiac scents proven to be a strong trigger for sexuality. The scents of essential oils can definitely contribute to your sexuality. These scents can also help in cases of impotence, anorgasmia, and weak erections. But bear in mind that the cause of the inability to have or keep an erection (impotence) or the inability to have an orgasm (anorgasmia) can be psychological and may not be solved simply by smelling a delightful scent.

Sexuality is supposed to create joy. Everything enhancing your joy makes your life richer and more beautiful. Having a healthy and fulfilling sex life will make you beautiful and radiant to others.

An aphrodisiac bath or body lotion can both delight us and ignite a delightful event. Aphrodisiac hip baths can strengthen the sexual organs and the capacity for erection or orgasm. They are recommended in cases of impotence or anorgasmia.

When selecting essential oils, you can choose between several aphrodisiac effects:

- To directly stimulate sexuality, use cardamom, cinnamon, coriander, black pepper, spruce, fir, and savory.
- To stimulate the hormones, use jasmine and sandalwood.
- To relax the mind, feel euphoric, and feel loving, use clary sage, neroli, patchouli, rose, and ylang-ylang.

- To strengthen an erection and the sexual organs in general, use ginger, ginseng, savory, fir, and juniper.
- As anaphrodisiacs (for calming sexuality), use marjoram and lavender.

Recipes for Enhancing Sexuality

Aphrodisiac Blend for the Aroma Lamp
5 drops patchouli, 2 sandalwood, 2 rose
or
4 drops ylang-ylang, 2 neroli, 1 bergamot
or
5 drops sandalwood, 2 jasmine

Aphrodisiac Bath
4 drops ylang-ylang, 2 sandalwood,
1 pepper, 1 cardamom
or
4 drops jasmine, 2 bergamot, 1 pepper
or
5 drops sandalwood, 1 jasmine, 3 cedarwood
(All these baths can be enriched
with honey and cream.)

Aphrodisiac Body Lotion
15 drops sandalwood, 2 jasmine,
4 ylang-ylang, 4 rose
(in 2 oz. vegetable oil)
or

5 drops ylang-ylang, 5 sandalwood,
5 patchouli, 5 rose
(in 2 oz. vegetable oil)

Hip Bath for Weak Erection, Impotence, or Anorgasmia
8 drops juniper or ginger, 2 sandalwood

10
Essential Oils for Women

For many women, the monthly period produces discomfort. In this chapter, I offer recipes for both the premenstrual phase and the menstrual phase of a woman's cycle.

Premenstrual Syndrome

Today, most of us are familiar with premenstrual syndrome, or PMS. During the premenstrual phase of a woman's cycle, the amount of liquid in the body increases as the body retains water. The lower abdomen and the breasts often swell. Mental concentration may be reduced. Women tend to be depressed or irritable. Exercise is a good way to improve mental and emotional symptoms as well as to release built-up liquids. Swimming is particularly good because of the healing effects of the water.

Essential oils that are effective in alleviating PMS include clary sage, geranium, and rose. Clary sage is especially important, as it has an all-around effect for all phases of the menstrual cycle. Baths, massages, and compresses with clary sage have been especially helpful to many women.

Water retention can be treated specifically with baths and massages containing the diuretic oils such as fennel, juniper, rosemary, and geranium.

To treat PMS with essential oils, you must use them consistently for one week before the onset of symptoms. Drinking a lot of fennel tea is also very helpful.

Mood swings, depression, and irritability can be balanced with the scents of clary sage, bergamot, jasmine, and rose. Using these oils in your baths, your body lotions, and your aroma lamp will help you to stay in a slightly euphoric, loving mood.

The Menstrual Period

The menstrual period is at times accompanied by headache or dizziness. These symptoms can be treated with Melissa or peppermint as a head compress, by inhalation, or in a bath. You can also use a dry inhalation (placing drops of the oil on a tissue and holding it under your nose) wherever you are, if you carry these oils with you during your period.

If your period is accompanied by cramps, pain, or gas, or is irregular, scanty, late, or lengthened, or if there is an extreme loss of blood or no blood at all (suspected pregnancy), you can use certain essential oils to combat the aches, cramps, and the irregular situation. A number of methods have been described in former chapters. I am going to list a few specific recipes for each method later on, but first here are the relevant oils for various conditions.

Irregular Period
clary sage, Melissa, rose

Late or Scanty Flow and Amenorrhea
basil, caraway, clary sage, cypress,
fennel, hyssop, juniper, lemongrass,
oregano, Melissa, myrrh, nutmeg,
Roman chamomile, rosemary, sage,
sassafras, pennyroyal, thyme

Cramps (Menstrual)
benzoin, bergamot, ginger, hyssop,
jasmine, peppermint, Roman chamomile,
rose, sage, sassafras

General Pain Release
anise, cajeput, carrot seed, clary sage,
cypress, juniper, lavender, marjoram,
Melissa, peppermint, Roman chamomile,
rose, sage, sassafras

Lengthened Period (Too Much Loss of Blood)
cinnamon, cypress, frankincense,
pennyroyal, rose

Uplifting the Mood
bergamot, clary sage, frankincense,
geranium, grapefruit, jasmine, lavender,
Melissa, orange, rose, rosewood,
tangerine, ylang-ylang

Hot hip baths, hot compresses, vaginal douches,
and aromatic tampons (see Chapter 5) are very effective in alleviating menstrual discomforts.

Pregnancy and Essential Oils

If you are pregnant, you should *never* use the following essential oils internally, and you should not use them externally in *high doses* as they may cause abortion: anise, basil, camphor, carrot seed, cinnamon, cedarwood, hyssop, marjoram, mint, myrrh, oregano, pennyroyal, sage, and thyme.

During the first three months of pregnancy, you should not take the following oils internally or in high doses in baths and massage: fennel, jasmine, peppermint, rose, and rosemary. These oils are said to be able to damage the fetus if taken in high doses and/or continuously.

In the first months of pregnancy, you can treat heartburn effectively with sandalwood taken internally. Low doses of geranium, lavender, frankincense, peppermint, and rose taken in a bath or with massage are generally helpful to the state of mood and the overall organism.

As the fetus grows, the mother-to-be's skin at the abdomen has to expand. A soft massage with lavender can prevent cracks in the connective tissue, which would otherwise remain after labor as stretch marks. The increasing weight the mother-to-be experiences as the fetus develops affects her legs and feet. They swell, ache, and tire faster than usual. Using rosemary and geranium in a massage oil is helpful. The mother-to-be's back is also stressed because it has to balance the body, which is now putting on weight in front. Massage the back with a blend of rosemary and lavender. Generally helpful for the skin, especially the breasts, is a body lotion with rose.

Childbirth

If this is a home birth, you can use compresses once you go into labor. Lavender and jasmine will deepen and strengthen the uterine contractions, while at the same time producing an analgesic effect. Jasmine also helps expel the afterbirth and helps the uterine muscles return to their former size.

Welcome the new baby to a room scented with a mild, pleasant smell, such as rose, jasmine, or bergamot. The baby will experience the birth and the first scent sensation as being more pleasant than the antiseptic, sterile odor of a hospital.

Menopause

Menopause changes a woman's hormonal balance. These hormonal changes cause hot flashes and are disorienting.

Fennel, geranium, Roman chamomile, sage, and cypress contain an estrogenlike substance and can help balance the hormones. Use these oils in aroma lamps, baths, and massages. Drinking similar herbal teas will also help with changes at menopause.

Gynecological Disorders

Disorders of the uterus can be treated with essential oils that tone and affect the uterus, such as clary sage, cypress, frankincense, jasmine, myrrh, parsley, and rose. All of these oils are equally beneficial, but parsley is especially helpful. They can be applied through compresses, massages, and baths.

Recipes for Women

PMS

PMS Bath (Diuretic)
6 drops rosemary, 4 juniper, 2 geranium

Menstrual Period Bath
(Uplifting Mood, Bringing on Period)
4 drops marjoram, 4 clary sage, 2 rose

Aroma Lamp Blend (Uplifting Mood)
2 drops rose, 2 bergamot, 2 jasmine
or
4 drops clary sage, 2 neroli

Internal Use (Nausea)
2 drops peppermint or Melissa or rose
(in a glass of water)

Late Period

Hip Bath
6 drops clary sage, 4 marjoram, 2 peppermint

Vaginal Douche
4 drops clary sage, 2 rose
(also for use with a tampon; see Chapter 5)

Hot Compress
4 drops clary sage, 4 marjoram, 2 peppermint

Lengthened Period (Blood Loss)

Hip Bath
5 drops cypress, 5 frankincense, 3 rose
(also for use with a tampon; see Chapter 5)

Vaginal Douche
3 drops cypress, 2 frankincense, 2 rose
(also for use with a tampon; see Chapter 5)

Hot Compress
4 drops cypress, 1 rose

11
Treating Children With Essential Oils

Children are born with a strong power to heal themselves. In addition, their young bodies haven't been exposed to as many years of toxic environment, unhealthy nutrition, and lack of movement as adults have.

When children go to school, however, they are exposed to the germs, bacteria, and viruses of the other children. Although this can become a troubling time of facing new diseases and discomforts, children's body systems are much more receptive to the benefits of essential oils.

Only very small doses should be administered with children. Never use as large a dose as mentioned so far in this book.

Roman chamomile and lavender are recommended for children. Both oils relieve pain, cramps, and spasms, and act as nerve sedatives. Use these oils in a highly diluted form in baths or body lotions, *but never give them internally.*

As the child becomes older, you can slowly increase the essential oil dosage. There is no exact age when a child turns into an adult. It depends on body constitution, growth, and psychological development.

As no human is exactly the same as another, I cannot give any accurate guidelines. The best advice is to try small doses and watch the results, increasing the dosage only in very small increments.

All children and teenagers have their own individual sensitivity. Usually, older children themselves know what they need. Let them smell the essential oil and tell you how it affects them. A last recommendation: *Keep all oils safely out of the reach of children!*

Recipes for Children

The doses in these recipes have been adjusted for children.

Pain-Relieving and Sleep-Inducing Bath
2 drops Roman chamomile, 2 lavender
(Mix with some vegetable oil.)

Skin-Care Bath
2 drops Roman chamomile, 1 rose
(Mix with 2 Tbsp. honey.)

Cold-Relief Bath
3 drops eucalyptus
(Mix with 2 Tbsp. honey.)

Cold or Flu
2 drops eucalyptus
(on the bed pillow)
or
4 drops eucalyptus or clary sage
(in the aroma lamp during the night)

Abdominal Cramps
2 drops Roman chamomile
(as hot compress)

Headache
2 drops Roman chamomile or lavender
(as cold compress)

Sleep and Relaxation
2 drops lavender
(on the bed pillow or in the aroma lamp)

Toothache, Earache
1 drop Roman chamomile
(as hot compress)
or
Roman chamomile
(Dab a diluted mix on the gums, or put a
cotton pad with Roman chamomile in the ear.)

Cough, Infection of the Respiratory System
2 drops eucalyptus or cypress
or hyssop or lavender
(Prepare with 2 pints of water for inhalation.
Support this treatment with 1 drop of the oil
on the bed pillow or some in the aroma lamp
at night, and a hot chest compress with lavender.)

Whooping Cough
2 drops eucalyptus, 1 basil, 1 hyssop
(Prepare with 2 pints of water for inhalation.)

Baby's Body Oil
3–5 drops rose or Roman chamomile
(Blend with 1 oz. carrier oil.)

12
Essential Oils and the Energy Centers (Chakras)

Scents and Spirituality

For six thousand years, different religions, sects, and esoteric schools—mostly in the East—have been experimenting with scents to determine their effects on spirituality. Scents have been used to help people relax, to deepen their breathing, to calm them emotionally, and to elevate them to a higher plane of being.

When we inhale natural scents, the spirit of the plant and our spirit meet. And who is to say that the being of a plant is lower than the human one? At the very least, plants have a consciousness and emotions, as has been proven by modern science.

Meditation is a key for the development of spirituality. When I meditate, I notice that certain scents make me calmer, more relaxed, and more sensitive, thereby enhancing my meditation. Mental and physical calm are essential to meditation, since what we are doing when we meditate is listening to our thoughts, feelings, and our inner selves.

The choice of the appropriate scent for meditation is an individual one; everyone responds differently to each scent. But after thousands of years of experimentation, certain guidelines can be given.

Many spiritual and esoteric schools speak of the diffferent bodies of human beings. Along with the physical body, there are also etheric, astral, and mental bodies. These bodies surround you like coats, each a specific distance from your physical body.

The etheric body receives the vital energy (also called chi, ki, or prana) that you need to live. The astral body receives the vibrations or emotions of other people. The mental body, which can be developed by any human during a lifetime, offers connection with the higher self and spiritual guidance. Some people see these bodies in various colors, called an aura.

Your physical body also has seven invisible energy centers, called chakras in the yogic tradition of India. They distribute the vital energy in the body and are located along the spine. Each chakra is responsible for specific systems and functions of the body, such as glands, emotions, and spiritual development. If all energy centers are in balance, energy is optimally distributed and you are healthy, vital, and complete. But the centers are frequently out of balance (especially in modern civilization) due to an overfunction or underfunction caused by a physical or emotional injury. The connected organs, systems, glands, emotions, and spirituality may be affected.

Essential Oils Recommended by the Sufis

The Sufis, a religious sect and esoteric school of the Middle East, mention the following essential oils as spiritual aids that work with the various chakras.

Amber (Styrax)

Amber, the "king of the scents" is closest to God. It is good for the heart center and helps with heart disorders. Wearing this scent will connect you with your spiritual body. Amber in the form of a pure, original oil, made from the resin of a tree, is rare. Pure amber oil has a strong, long-lasting scent.

Frankincense

Frankincense is used to cleanse the aura, to enhance deep, relaxed breathing, and to create a feeling of space and clarity. It expands the consciousness and is a preferred scent for meditation.

Musk (Ambretta)

The Sufis use musk for disorders of the heart, sexual problems, and low vitality (second-chakra issues). When you smell musk, you will understand why it is considered an aphrodisiac.

Myrrh

Used to calm, cleanse, and heal the physical body, myrrh works well in meditation blends.

Rose

Called the "mother of the scents," rose cleanses all the bodies (physical, etheric, astral, and mental) and encourages the consciousness to reach higher levels. Without a doubt, it is the most important heart scent and is used to awaken the fourth chakra through love, compassion, friendship, and openness.

Sandalwood
The scent of sandalwood calms rough emotions (the ego). It is good for issues of the third chakra, and it stimulates the first and seventh chakras as well.

The Chakras and Related Essential Oils

First Chakra

The first energy center is called the "root chakra" and is located at the base of the spinal column between the anus and the genitals. This chakra rules the kidneys, legs, feet, genitals, anus, spine, nerves, and skin (dermis). It is the site of the will to live, the survival mechanisms, kundalini or life energy, and grounding to the earth. Related essential oils include cinnamon, clove, nutmeg, pepper, and sandalwood.

Second Chakra

The second energy center is known as the "sacral chakra" and is located a distance of four fingers' width under the navel in the middle of the lower abdomen. This chakra rules the sexual instinct, reproduction, and vitality. Related organs are the ovaries, testes, uterus, reproductive organs, abdomen, pelvis, and lumbar vertebra. Related essential oils include ginseng, musk, sandalwood, and ylang-ylang.

Third Chakra

The third energy center is called the "solar plexus chakra" and is located below the shoulder blades in the central, stomach region of the body. This chakra deals with rough emotions, the ego's self-interest, and personal power. It rules the liver, gallbladder, stomach, intestines, sympathetic nervous system, abdominal viscera, pancreas, and diaphragm. Dysfunction may cause cancer, digestive problems, skin problems, negativity, and disharmony. Related essential oils include ginger, lemon, rosemary, sage, and thyme.

Fourth Chakra

Called the "heart chakra," the fourth energy center is located at the dorsal spine behind the heart. It is responsible for love, compassion, friendship, group consciousness, and joy. It rules the heart, blood circulation, lower lungs, breasts, breast vertebrae, immune system, thymus gland, and vagus nerve. Related essential oils include neroli, petitgrain, rose, and rosewood.

Fifth Chakra

The fifth energy center is called the "throat chakra" and is located at the base of the throat. It governs creativity, visions, fantasy, communication, and expression. It rules the vocal area, respiratory tract, digestive tract, throat, arms, hands, and the thyroid and parathyroid glands. This center connects mind and emotions. Related essential oils include bergamot, frankincense, geranium, and jasmine.

Sixth Chakra

Called the "brow chakra" or "third eye," the sixth energy center is located in the middle of the forehead between the eyebrows. It is the seat of intuition, intellect, higher mental clairvoyance, and higher wisdom disconnected from the ego. This third eye enables you to "see clearly," uninfluenced by prejudice and emotions. It rules the forehead, ears, nose, teeth, lower brain stem, pituitary gland, and nervous system. Related essential oils include cajeput, cedarwood, eucalyptus, juniper, and peppermint.

Seventh Chakra

The seventh energy center is called the "crown chakra" and is located at the top of the head. The seat of the spiritual "will to be," it possesses blueprints of all the energy centers and is the connective center between humans and the world of divine spirit. It balances the personal will with the love of God. It governs the brain, central nervous system, cerebral cortex, and pineal gland. Related essential oils include amber, blue chamomile, lavender, myrrh, and rose.

There are several suppliers offering essential oils with pleasant scents that may be effective with the seven chakras. By smelling the scents, you can begin to determine the ingredients. Remember, not all people have identical vibrations. You might react to different oils than your friends. Find your own individual blend. Trusting your intuition—being able to "feel" the oils—will tell you what blend is best for you.

When applying essential oils (prepared like massage oils; see Chapter 5), you should create a quiet, meditative atmosphere at home. Light some candles, play soothing music, and lie or sit in a relaxed position. Massage the oil with the right hand on the site of the chakra and mentally focus on this area. Clockwise circular movements work best. Use your imagination to visualize what you want the energy center to be or to do. Imagine the center opening the way a flower opens its petals, with its energy flowing and harmony spreading all over the area, the related organs, and so forth. Work with a particular center for one week daily, and then change to another one.

13
Essential Oils and Astrology

In former times, teachers of astrology assigned various plants, herbs, trees, and flowers to particular planets based on their color, form, content, and the location where they grew. In the Middle Ages, astrology of the plant world provided important guidance for the doctor who was deciding upon a particular prescription for a particular patient.

This astrological assignment of plants provided the guidelines for the assignment of the essential oils derived from them. Each scent has particular astrological aspects. Western astrology and Chinese medicine both refer to four basic elements—earth, air, fire, and water.

If you use essential oils in connection with their astrological applications, you may be able to balance your elements. For example, if you have many planets in the element "air" in your horoscope, you may experience yourself as airy, ungrounded, or unrealistic. In this case, you may need an earthy scent to balance you, ground you, and make you more realistic.

While space prevents me from an in-depth discussion, I will briefly describe how to use scents to balance the elements in your astrological chart.

Balancing Elements With Scents

Lack of Fire

A lack of fire can result in low self-esteem, a lack of enthusiasm, avoidance of challenges, no joy of life, no trust in life, and lack of initiative. Balance this with fiery scents such as cinnamon, myrrh, neroli, and orange.

Too Much Fire

Too much fire can result in overactivity, restlessness, being too impulsive, having too little compassion, and carelessness. Balance this with watery scents such as chamomile, fennel, jasmine, and myrtle.

Lack of Water

A lack of water can result in having little connection to your emotions and feelings, difficulties in dealing with others' emotions, less trust in your own intuition, and a tendency to rationalize everything. Balance this with watery scents such as chamomile, fennel, jasmine, and myrtle.

Too Much Water

Too much water can result in an unbalanced relationship between emotions and their triggers, being overly emotional, an inability to cope with everyday life, pulling back from difficulties, and avoidance of challenges. Positive attributes include an enormous disposition for love, compassion, helpfulness, and high sensitivity. Balance this with fiery scents such as cinnamon, myrrh, neroli, and orange.

Lack of Earth

A lack of earth can result in an unrealistic outlook; carelessness concerning money, work, nutrition, house, and family; and avoidance of responsibility. Positive attributes include unlimited creativity, imagination, and high spiritual potential. Balance this with earthy scents such as basil, cedarwood, musk, patchouli, and sandalwood.

Too Much Earth

Too much earth can result in a lack of imagination, a lack of vision, intolerance, being overly practical and efficient, and too little joy in life. Balance this with airy scents such as bergamot, grapefruit, lavender, mint, and orange.

Lack of Air

A lack of air can result in a highly materialistic person with no perspective on everyday life. Each emotion and action is overemphasized; there is no openness to the new and the unexpected. A lack of air also results in being critical. Balance with airy scents such as bergamot, grapefruit, lavender, mint, and orange.

Too Much Air

Too much air can result in too much thinking and planning, a lack of sponteneity, a lack of relationship to reality, dreaminess, hyperactivity, oversensitivity, and a lack of distance from work. Positive attributes include originality, creativity, good organizing skills, and the ability to socialize with different people. Balance this with earthy scents such as basil, cedarwood, musk, patchouli, and sandalwood.

Planet Relationships

Sun
benzoin, bergamot, frankincense, myrrh,
neroli, orange, patchouli, rosemary, tangerine

Moon
chamomile

Mars
basil, coriander, garlic, onion,
pepper, sage, tarragon

Venus
geranium, lily of the valley, neroli,
rose, thyme, verena, ylang-ylang

Mercury
carrot seed, clary sage, fennel,
lavender, marjoram

Saturn
camphor, cypress, eucalyptus, frankincense, pine

Jupiter
anise, clove, coriander, jasmine,
juniper, Melissa, sage

Uranus
cedarwood, sandalwood

Star Sign Relationships

Aries	ginger, rosemary
Taurus	marjoram, thyme
Gemini	clary sage, verbena
Cancer	hyssop, jasmine, Melissa
Leo	chamomile, orange
Virgo	fennel, lavender, peppermint
Libra	lily of the valley, neroli, rose, thyme, ylang-ylang
Scorpio	basil, coriander, garlic, tarragon
Sagittarius	cedarwood, Melissa, sage
Capricorn	cypress, pine
Aquarius	frankincense, myrtle, mimosa
Pisces	clove, cinnamon, sandalwood

The information in this chapter does not include all the essential oils mentioned in this book, as not all plants have been assigned to planets or signs. There is also some confusion in the literature concerning the assignments. My advice is to follow your feelings, and trust your nose!

14
Cooking With Essential Oils

You might have detected in the preceding chapters several essential oils whose names are also known in the kitchen.

Natural and pure essential oils are not only healing agents but also highly concentrated spices. But remember that essential oils should be used only in very small amounts in cooking. They are best added after cooking or boiling so the scent doesn't evaporate. Dissolve the essential oils with the common carrier oils and stir everything well.

Essential oils are highly concentrated; you will need only one to two drops in an average meal for four people. Here are some examples of particular dishes, sauces, dressings, and drinks prepared with essential oils:

- Season Italian meals with basil, garlic, marjoram, oregano, sage, or thyme essential oils, diluted in cream or vegetable oil.
- Season mayonnaise with garlic essence.
- Season salad dressing with basil, garlic, parsley, lemon, or peppermint essential oils.
- Season salad oils with basil, garlic, rosemary, or savory essential oils.

- Season cakes with lemon, orange, or vanilla essential oils; dilute the oils in honey.
- Season desserts with grapefruit, orange, or tangerine essential oils.
- Season sauces with basil, marjoram, or sage essential oils; dilute the oils in vegetable oil.
- Use vanilla essence in dessert sauces.
- Flavor vegetables with dill, fennel, and savory essential oils; dilute the oils in boiling or steaming water.
- Make aromatic cold drinks with bergamot, lemon, orange, and tangerine essential oils.
- Make aromatic teas with bergamot, fennel, jasmine, peppermint, rose, or sage essential oils. Drip essential oils in regular black tea or herb tea, shake well, and let the tea stand to blend well. (Earl Grey tea is black tea leaves with bergamot!)
- Make aromatic honey with lavender, orange, Melissa, or tangerine essential oils; heat up the honey until it becomes liquid and stir in the essential oil.

15
Using Essential Oils
Around the House

Several essential oils provide effective alternatives to commercial scents to use around the house. For example, rather than using commercial fabric softeners for their smell, scent the wash load with two drops of lavender in the rinse water. Or scent your dishwashing detergent with natural, antiseptic lemon oil (usually, commercial detergents with a lemon scent contain mostly *synthetic* lemon).

To cleanse your kitchen counters, floors, or bath tiles, add a few drops of antiseptic, pleasant-smelling essential oils to your cleanser and water, such as lemon, lavender, or peppermint. If you prefer the scent of an orchard, use orange, tangerine, or grapefruit. Or if the woods are your favorite habitat, use a blend of fir, pine, and one to two drops of cedarwood. This blend is very helpful if you or somebody else in your house has an infectious illness, such as a cold or the flu.

Other possible household applications of essential oils include spraying your laundry before ironing, placing a cotton handkerchief in your dryer, or spraying your closets with a pleasant scent. Oils with a high scent intensity and slow evaporation rate are amber, cedarwood, geranium, jasmine, lavender, rose, sandal-wood, and ylang-ylang. Their scents will have staying power in your closet. I spray my whole closet and clothes regularly with a dilution of two pints of water and twenty drops of sandalwood. It is such a joy to get some good-smelling shirts or underwear out of the closet or bureau in the morning!

Rather than synthetic, chemical scents in a sauna, you can use the natural aromas of essential oils, which benefit the respiratory system and the immune system. You can use eucalyptus, fir, sage, thyme, cedarwood, pine, or lemon. These oils are antiseptic and have an excellent anti-infectious effect. Using oils in the sauna is especially important if you are sharing it with many people. In wintertime, when many people have colds and flus, essential oils can help prevent the spread of viruses and bacteria in the sauna's air.

You can deter bugs, such as mosquitoes, moths, and flies, with insect repellent oils; these can be used either in the aroma lamp or in a special body oil. Effective repellent oils are basil, cedarwood, citronella, clove, cypress, eucalyptus, geranium, lemongrass, Melissa, and peppermint. Even rats and mice will avoid your house if you spray eucalyptus (blended with water) in your basement. (Use one pint of water with five drops of essential oil to make a "spray.")

16
Restrictions on the Use of Essential Oils

If you are using essential oils without the advice of an aromatherapist but closely follow the recipes mentioned in this book, you are not going to be endangered by toxicity or side effects. *But you must pay close attention to the following restrictions.* The following oils should be used in low doses or not at all.

Skin Irritants

Use up to three drops in baths, and a maximum of five drops with two ounces of carrier oil in massage oils and body oils. Be careful in using these essential oils, especially with sensitive skin.

basil	lemongrass
cajeput	Melissa
camphor	nutmeg
caraway	pennyroyal
cardamom	pepper
clove	peppermint
coriander	sage
eucalyptus	thyme
lemon	verbena

Essential Oils to Avoid During Pregnancy

Never use the following essential oils internally or in high doses in baths or massage oils, as they may cause abortion.

basil	marjoram
camphor	myrrh
caraway	nutmeg
carrot	oregano
cedarwood	pennyroyal
clove	peppermint
hyssop	rosemary
frankincense	sage
juniper	sassfras

High Blood Pressure

Never use the following essential oils internally. Use only low doses in baths, body oils, or massage oils.

hyssop	thyme
rosemary	tuja
sage	

Toxic Doses of Essential Oils

The following essential oils are toxic if more than ten drops are taken internally at one time.

anise	cinnamon
camphor	clove
cedarwood	fennel

hyssop	pennyroyal
lemon	pine
nutmeg	sage
oregano	

Children

Never give babies and young children the same dose of essential oils as adults. Only in rare situations give children essential oils internally (for these exceptions, see Chapter 11).

Epilepsy

If you have a history of epilepsy, never take the following oils internally. Use them only in very low doses in baths, body oils, massage oils, and by inhalation.

hyssop	sage
fennel	tuja

Homeopathic Treatment and Essential Oils

Homeopathic remedies and essential oils should not be used as a cure at the same time. Occasional aromatic baths, and use of the aroma lamp and cosmetics made with essential oils will not interfere with homeopathic treatment. Of the various essential oils, camphor and peppermint especially interfere with homeopathy.

17
Index of Essential Oils:
Properties, Uses, and Hints

The following oils will be described:

Amber (Styrax)
Angelica Root
Anise
Arnica
Basil
Bay
Benzoin
Bergamot
Birch
Cajeput
Camphor
Caraway
Cardamom
Carrot Seed
Cedarwood
Chamomile, Blue
    and Roman
Cinnamon
Citronella
Clary Sage
Clove
Coriander

Cumin
Cypress
Eucalyptus
Fennel, Sweet
Fir
Frankincense
Galbanum
Garlic
Geranium
Ginger
Grapefruit
Hyssop
Immortelle
Jasmine
Juniper
Lavender
Lemon
Lemongrass
Marjoram
Melissa (Balm,
    Lemon Balm)
Mimosa

Myrrh
Myrtle
Neroli (Orange
  Blossom)
Niaouli
Nutmeg
Onion
Orange
Oregano
Parsley
Patchouli
Pennyroyal
Pepper, Black
Peppermint
Petitgrain
Pine, Mountain
Pine, Stone
Rose

Rosemary
Rosewood
Sage
Sandalwood
Sassafras
Savory
Tangerine
Tarragon
Tea Tree
Thyme
Tuberose
Tuja
Turpentine
Verbena
Vetiver
Violet, Blue
Ylang-ylang

Amber (Styrax)

Latin name: Liquidambar orientalis
Obtained from: The bark and resin of the tree
Scent: slightly sweet, erogenous, musky
Properties: Cleanses the aura; harmonizes the electromagnetic body; slightly aphrodisiac; acts as nerve sedative.
General uses: Treats nervousness, overexcitement; promotes meditation.
Hints: You will rarely find original amber oil. Most of the oils offered and most of the amber "stones" available in stores are blends of several other oils that result in a similar scent.

Angelica Root
Latin name: Angelica archangelica
Obtained from: Primarily the roots, also from the leaves and seeds
Scent: Earthy, slightly musky, pepperlike, aromatic
Properties: Acts as stomach tonic; aids digestion; removes mucus from respiratory tract; strengthens immune system; acts as stimulant, fungicide, bactericide, antiseptic, nerve sedative.
General uses: Treats digestive problems, all internal infections, and nervousness.

Anise
Latin name: Pimpinella anisum
Obtained from: The whole plant and the seed
Scent: Sweet, herblike, similar to licorice
Properties: Acts as body stimulant, stomach tonic; relieves spasms; acts as antiseptic, narcotic.
General uses: Treats migraines, fainting, digestive problems, flatulence, vomiting, menstrual cramps, colics, asthma, cough, impotence, and anorgasmia.
Hints: Do not take high doses internally or use on a long-term basis as damage to stomach mucous membrane, brain cells, and kidneys may result. The occasional use of low doses in baths, compresses, or aroma lamps is fine.

Arnica
Latin name: Arnica montana
Obtained from: The roots and flowers of the plant
Scent: Earthy, herblike, slightly woody
Properties: Acts as body stimulant, diuretic, deodor-

ant; benefits skin; heals wounds; promotes the formation of scar tissue.

Skin and hair: Treats cellulite, body odor, cracked and chapped skin, wounds, cuts, burns, sores.

Hints: Difficult to find in the form of an essential oil. The extract of the plant in a carrier oil is easier to find and is very good for skin care and healing.

Basil

Latin name: Ocimum basilicum
Obtained from: The whole herb
Scent: Penetrating, sweet, spicy, fresh, aniselike
Properties: Relieves spasms; acts as stomach tonic; aids digestion; acts as nerve tonic and sedative, body tonic, antiseptic; stimulates menstrual flow; removes mucus from respiratory tract; acts as abortive agent; beneficial to skin; acts as insect repellent.

General uses: Treats bronchitis, whooping cough, flu, colds, fever, digestive problems, vomiting, nausea, lack of or scanty menstruation, nervousness.

Skin and hair: Acts as skin toner, facial cleanser; treats congested skin.

Emotions and mind: Treats mental fatigue and confusion; regenerates mental powers; treats depression, anxiety, apathy, PMS, insomnia.

Hints: Irritates sensitive skin if high doses are used. Causes hot-cold sensation in bath. Contraindicated during pregnancy. Acts as insect repellent.

Bay

Latin name: Pimenta acris, racemosa

Obtained from: The leaves of the tree
Scent: Strong, sharp, clovelike
Properties: Acts as body stimulant, antiseptic, nerve tonic; benefits hair.
General uses: Treats weakness of circulation, colds, flu.
Skin and hair: Helps with nail and hair care, hair loss.

Benzoin
Latin name: Styrax benzoin
Obtained from: The resin of the storax tree
Scent: Sweet, like raisins, balmy, warm
Properties: Removes mucus from respiratory tract; acts as antiseptic; relieves spasms; acts as diuretic, heart tonic, deodorant, antidepressant; benefits skin; acts as anti-inflammatory agent.
General uses: Treats colds, coughs, bronchitis, asthma, bladder infection, infection of sexual organs, colics, arthritis, gout, gonorrhea, vaginal discharge.
Skin and hair: Relieves bruises, irritation and inflammation of skin, body odor, sores.
Emotions and mind: Treats emotional exhaustion, overexcitement, sorrow; helps create distance from life's strains.
Hints: Recommended for preservation of cosmetics as it is very effective and has a pleasant scent.

Bergamot
Latin name: Citrus auranthium
Obtained from: The peel of the bitter orange
Scent: Fresh, fruity, sweet, distinct
Properties: Strongly antiseptic; acts as antidepressant;

relieves pain, spasms; removes mucus from respiratory system; aids digestion; expels intestinal worms; acts as deodorant, antidepressant; benefits skin; acts as tanning agent; heals wounds; aids in the formation of scar tissue.

General uses: Treats infections of respiratory system, mouth, tonsils, urinary tract, bladder; treats colds, diphtheria, colics, flatulence, digestive disorders, gallstones, fever, gonorrhea, vaginal discharge, herpes of genitals or mouth, vaginal itching, intestinal worms.

Skin and hair: Excellent in treating all types of skin, acne, blemished skin, eczema, scabies, abscesses, varicose veins, wounds, cuts, sores, burns, ulcers, body odor, bad breath; acts as suntan oil.

Emotions and mind: Treats depression, anxiety, stress, nervous tension, PMS, insomnia; scent is cheerful.

Hints: Very useful for bath oils, body oils, facial cosmetics. Can be used for suntan oils or creams but has to be used carefully as the *oil can cause dark spots* (which usually disappear after some days) with intense sunshine or when exposing the skin to sun at high elevations. This effect is true of all citrus oils (lemon, orange, tangerine, grapefruit). This oil gives the famous Earl Grey tea its aroma.

Birch

Latin name: Betula lenta
Obtained from: The bark and branches of the tree
Scent: Leathery, balsamic
Properties: Acts as antiseptic, anti-inflammatory agent, antitoxic, body stimulant; benefits hair.

General uses: Treats rheumatism, sore muscles, blood toxification, tendonitis.

Skin and hair: Treats ulcers, rash, cellulite, hair loss, skin inflammation.

Cajeput

Latin name: Melaleuca leucodendron

Obtained from: The leaves and twigs of the tree

Scent: Strongly herblike, similar to eucalyptus

Properties: Acts as antiseptic; removes mucus from respiratory system; relieves pain; acts as bactericide, anti-inflammatory agent; eases grippy pains; expels gas; acts as body stimulant and tonic; benefits skin and hair.

General uses: Treats infections of respiratory system, colds, flu, inflammation of mucous membrane, sinusitis; treats aches of head, teeth, and throat; treats arthritis, sore muscles, general weakness and fatigue of the body, tumors.

Skin and hair: Treats skin inflammation, hair loss; helps with bald head care.

Emotions and mind: Treats apathy, inactivity, mental fatigue; scent is very stimulating for the mind and the body.

Hints: Possible irritation of skin if high doses are used in bath oil, body oil, or facial oil. Use niauoli oil as a substitute.

Camphor

Latin name: Cinnamonum camphora

Obtained from: The juice of the tree

Scent: Medicinal, strong, fresh, eucalyptuslike

Properties: Acts as heart tonic, respiratory and circulation tonic and stimulant, nerve sedative; acts to cool and warm; aids digestion; acts as antiseptic; provides pain relief, spasm relief; eases grippy pains; expels gas; acts as bowel-evacuation stimulant, diuretic; heals wounds; raises blood pressure; acts as antidepressant; benefits skin.

General uses: Treats physical weakness, weak heart, psychosomatic and nervous ailments, bronchitis, colds, flu, fever, pneumonia, digestive and intestinal troubles, vomiting, rheumatism, gout, fungal infections, irritation of the genitals, low blood pressure.

Skin and hair: Treats acne, blemished skin, bruises, sprains, wounds, cuts, sores; stimulates skin metabolism; helps with general skin care; cools and warms skin.

Emotions and mind: Stimulates when depressed; calms when overexcited, annoyed, or experiencing insomnia.

Hints: Irritation and redness of skin is possible if high doses are used in bath oil, body oil, or facial oil. High doses taken internally are toxic.

Caraway

Latin name: Carum carvi
Obtained from: The fruit and leaves of the herb
Scent: Strongly herblike, typically carawaylike
Properties: Acts as body tonic, stomach tonic, diuretic; provides spasm relief; stimulates appetite, menstrual flow; acts as abortive agent.
General uses: Treats nervous digestion troubles, stom-

ach cramps, flatulence, appetite loss, hiccups, intestinal congestion, constipation, heart flutter or rush (palpitation), lack of or scanty and painful menstruation (amenorrhea), heavy menstrual cramps.

Hints: Contraindicated during pregnancy. May irritate skin in bath oil, body oil, or facial oil if high doses are used.

Cardamom

Latin name: Elettaria cardamomum

Obtained from: The seeds of the herb

Scent: Spicy, strong, aromatic, balsamic, slightly flowery

Properties: Aids digestion; acts as stomach tonic, mind tonic, antiseptic, aphrodisiac, diuretic, appetite stimulant; relieves spasms.

General uses: Treats digestive problems, appetite loss, weak stomach, heartburn, flatulence, nausea, vomiting, colic, spasms, pain in lower abdomen, coughs, physical weakness, slow metabolism, impotence, and anorgasmia.

Emotions and mind: Treats mental fatigue, mental confusion. Scent acts to clear the mind.

Hints: May irritate skin in bath oil, body oil, or facial oil if high doses are used. A stimulating, aphrodisiac oil. Refreshing as a bath oil.

Carrot Seed

Latin name: Daucus carota

Obtained from: The plant's seed

Scent: Woody and earthy, slightly erogenous

Properties: Acts as internal cleanser, liver and gall tonic; stimulates menstrual flow; benefits skin; acts as abortive agent.

General uses: Treats hepatitis, gall and liver insufficiency, absence of or scanty menstrual flow, menstrual cramps.

Skin and hair: Helps with general skin care, skin nutrition; acts as tanning agent; benefits both dry and oily skin; treats blemished skin.

Emotions and mind: Treats overexcitement, nervousness; scent has slightly aphrodisiac effects on the mind.

Hints: Contraindicated during pregnancy.

Cedarwood

Latin name: Cedrus atlantica
Obtained from: The twigs and wood of the tree
Scent: Harmonious sweet-sour, woody
Properties: Benefits skin and hair; removes mucus from respiratory tract; benefits bladder; acts as diuretic, antiseptic, antidepressant, insect repellent; calms; acts as abortive agent.

General uses: Treats flu, bronchitis, bladder infection, bladder pain, pyelitis (infection of the pelvis of the kidneys), gonorrhea.

Skin and hair: Helps with general skin care, skin inflammation, acne, blemished skin, eczema, general hair care, oily hair, dandruff.

Emotions and mind: Treats depression, anxiety.

Hints: Contraindicated during pregnancy. May irritate skin in bath oil, body oil, or facial oil if high doses are used. Acts as insect repellent (especially for moths). Preferred scent for men's facial cosmetics.

Chamomile, Blue and Roman

Latin names:
  Blue   chamomile = *Matricaria   chamomilla*
  Roman chamomile = *Anthemis nobilis*
Obtained from: The flowers of the herb (blue chamomile); the flowers and leaves of the herb (Roman chamomile)
Scents: Strong, herblike, sweet (blue chamomile); fruity, sweet, like leaves fermenting in fall (Roman chamomile)
Properties: Acts as anti-inflammatory agent, stomach tonic, antidepressant, anticonvulsive, antiseptic; eases grippy pains; relieves pain, spasms; expels gas; acts as nerve sedative, diuretic; stimulates menstrual flow; reduces fever; acts as nerve tonic, liver tonic; heals wounds.
General uses: Treats conjunctivitis, burning or tired eyes, headaches; treats aches in the eyes, teeth, ears, nerves, stomach, and intestines; treats migraine, menstrual cramps, excessive menstrual bleeding, gingivitis, colitis, anemia, allergies, diarrhea, dyspepsia, flatulence, vomiting, gastralgia, gastritis, neuralgia, rheumatism, peptic ulcers, teething pains, urinary stones, vaginitis, vulvar pruritus (itching of vagina), colic, jaundice, fever, nervousness.
Skin and hair: Helps with general skin care; treats skin inflammation, dermatitis, skin aches, sunburn, acne, blemished skin, wounds, cuts, sores,

rash; helps with hair care for blond hair.

Emotions and mind: Treats irritability, depression, hysteria, insomnia; calms nerves, mind, and emotions.

Hints: Blue chamomile is especially valuable for inflammations because of its high content of azulen, which gives the oil its blue color. Roman chamomile is particularly useful for children, since its effects are mild and it is nontoxic. It is very calming (in bath and body oils), and acts as an excellent pain reliever and skin remedy (for scratches, bruises, wounds, and chapped or dry skin).

Cinnamon

Latin name: Cinnamomum ceylanicum

Obtained from: The bark or the leaves of the tree

Scent: The scent of the leaves' oil is warm, spicy, clovelike; the scent of the bark's oil is warm, spicy-sweet, but stronger than the leaves' oil.

Properties: Acts as strong antiseptic, antiputrefactive; aids digestion; acts as aphrodisiac; arrests bleeding; benefits skin; acts as heart tonic; relieves spasms; acts as abortive agent.

General uses: Treats physical weakness, colds, flu, cough, bronchitis, digestive problems, weak stomach, flatulence, diarrhea, intestinal cramps, putrefaction in the intestines, absence of or scanty menstrual flow, excessive menstrual bleeding, bleeding wounds, impotence and anorgasmia.

Skin and hair: Helps with skin care for lifeless or sallow skin; acts as after-shave; treats scabies and lice.

Hints: Contraindicated during pregnancy. Possible irritation of skin if high doses are used in bath oil, body oil, or facial oil. Toxic if high doses are taken internally. No internal use recommended. Acts as good air freshener in aroma lamp (blend with bergamot).

Citronella

Latin name: Cymbopogon nardus
Obtained from: The grass
Scent: Roselike, sweet, woody, flowery
Properties: Stimulate body and mind; refreshes; acts as fungicide, antiseptic, bactericide.
General uses: Treats rheumatism, fungal skin infections.
Hints: Traditional insect repellent (for mosquitoes) used in Asian countries; acts as air freshener; disliked by cats and rats. Possible allergic reactions if used in body oil or bath oil.

Clary Sage

Latin name: Salvia sclarea
Obtained from: The blossoming herb
Scent: Light, haylike, warm, sweet, amberlike
Properties: Acts as nerve sedative, euphoric, body tonic; relieves spasms; acts as antiseptic, aphrodisiac, nerve tonic; stimulates menstrual flow; raises blood pressure; acts as deodorant; helps with skin and hair care; acts as anti-inflammatory agent.
General uses: Treats conjunctivitis, throat infections, nerve ailments, digestive troubles, flatulence,

stomach aches, intestinal cramps, kidney disorders, low blood pressure, absence of or scanty menstrual flow, menstrual cramps, vaginal discharge, impotence and anorgasmia, nervousness.

Skin and hair: Helps with general skin care; treats skin inflammation, ulcers, boils, heavy sweating; helps with general hair care; treats dandruff, hair loss.

Emotions and mind: Treats depression, nervous and emotional tension, negativity, grief, anxiety, PMS, lack of inspiration; scent makes one euphoric.

Hints: Contraindicated during pregnancy. Not to be used with alcoholic beverages. Used as an alternative to sage because of its milder effects.

Clove

Latin name: Suzygium aromaticum
Obtained from: The buds or leaves of the tree
Scent: Strong, warm, sweet, spicy
Properties: Acts as strong antiseptic, insect repellent, body tonic; relieves pain, spasms; benefits skin; acts as abortive agent.

General uses: Treats toothaches, gum infections; helps with gum care; aids digestive problems; treats diarrhea, flatulence, absence of or scanty menstrual flow; helps with regeneration after illness.

Skin and hair: Treats warts, ulcers, scrapes, scabies, pussing wounds; disinfects wounds; treats insect bites, calluses; acts as after-shave.

Emotions and mind: Treats mental fatigue, loss of concentration.

Hints: Toxic and caustic, therefore to be used only

in small doses. Possible irritation of skin if high doses are used in bath oil, body oil, or facial oil. Acts as effective disinfectant for air, floor, kitchen, bath, toilets. Contraindicated during pregnancy. Warming, vitalizing, and soothing scent for wintertime (blend with clove, cinnamon, and nutmeg).

Coriander
Latin name: Coriandrum sativum
Obtained from: The dry seeds of the herb
Scent: Fruity, aromatic, light
Properties: Acts as body tonic, stomach tonic, nerve tonic; aids digestion; stimulates appetite; relieves pain; warms; acts as aphrodisiac; stimulates menstrual flow; acts as abortive agent.
General uses: Treats digestive problems, stomach and intestinal cramps, flatulence, appetite loss, nerve aches, rheumatism, impotence and anorgasmia, general physical and nerve weakness, nervousness, absence of or scanty menstrual flow, menstrual cramps; helps with regeneration after illness.
Emotions and mind: Treats shock, anxiety, irritability, mental fatigue.
Hints: Contraindicated during pregnancy.

Cumin
Latin name: Cuminum cyminum
Obtained from: The plant's seed
Scent: Slightly sweet, powdery, spicy
Properties: Acts as stomach tonic; aids digestion; relieves spasms; stimulates appetite.

General uses: Treats digestive problems, appetite loss, stomach and intestinal cramps, flatulence, diarrhea, slow circulation, weak heart.

Hints: Related to coriander, ingredient of curry.

Cypress

Latin name: Cupressus sempervirens

Obtained from: The leaves and twigs of the tree

Scent: Fresh, dry, warm, amberlike, aromatic, smoky

Properties: Arrests bleeding; acts as uterus tonic; causes constriction of capillaries; acts as deodorant, astringent, liver tonic, diuretic, nerve sedative, antiseptic; relieves spasms; benefits skin.

General uses: Treats gum bleeding, asthma, whooping cough, spasmodic cough, coughing up blood, diarrhea, liver disorders, influenza, rheumatism, nervous tension, internal bleeding, hemorrhoids, varicose veins, bed-wetting, pus, menopausal problems, nervousness.

Skin and hair: Treats oily skin, varicose veins, cellulite, body odor, foot odor.

Emotions and mind: Treats restlessness, irritability.

Hints: Works as refreshing, relaxing bath oil. Acts as good insect repellent.

Eucalyptus

Latin name: Eucalyptus globulus, others

Obtained from: The leaves and young twigs of the tree

Scent: Fresh, medicinal, pungent, camphorlike (*eucalyptus citriodora*—lemon and roselike)

Properties: Removes mucus from respiratory tract;

acts as antiseptic; reduces fever; relieves spasms; acts as hypoglycemic, stomach tonic, stimulant, diuretic, deodorant; heals wounds; aids in the formation of scar tissue; reduces fever; acts as disinfectant, insect repellent; benefits skin; stimulates mind.

General uses: Treats colds, flu, bronchitis, coughs, inflammation of the mucous membrane, asthma, tuberculosis, sinusitis, throat infections, migraine, digestive problems, diarrhea, diphtheria, dyspepsia, malaria, cholera, neuralgia, gallstones, urinary tract infections, fever, herpes, vaginal discharge, gonorrhea, rheumatism, hemorrhage, diabetes, nephritis (kidneys), scarlet fever.

Skin and hair: Acts as skin cleanser; treats wounds, cuts, sores, blisters, ulcers.

Emotions and mind: Treats lack of concentration, mental irritation; scent creates a feeling of space.

Hints: Possible irritation of skin if high doses are used in bath oil, body oil, or facial oil. Recommended for disinfecting air and items if infectious diseases are present. Acts as insect repellent; also repels mice and cockroaches.

Fennel, Sweet
Latin name: Foeniculum vulgare dulce
Obtained from: The seeds (fruits) of the herb
Scent: Warm, sweet, aniselike
Properties: Aids digestion; acts as stomach tonic; eases grippy pains; expels gas; acts as antiseptic; relieves spasms; acts as diuretic, tonic; stimulates menstrual flow; removes mucus from respiratory

tract; stimulates bowel evacuation; expels intestinal worms; detoxifies; balances appetite; benefits skin.

General uses: Treats digestive problems, flatulence, constipation, dyspepsia, hiccups, colic, gallstones, absence of or scanty menstrual flow, menstrual cramps, menopausal problems (oil contains estrogenlike substances); detoxifies (from alcohol overdose); treats overeating; stimulates liver and spleen.

Skin and hair: Helps with general skin care; treats cellulite.

Emotions and mind: Treats overexcitement, restlessness; scent makes one cautious, loving, and calm.

Hints: Has mild effects on body and emotions. Reduces hunger; good for fasts and diets.

Fir

Latin name: Picea abies
Obtained from: The needles of the tree
Scent: Fresh, light, spicy
Properties: Acts as antiseptic, body tonic, deodorant, aphrodisiac.

General uses: Treats colds, coughs, flu, bronchitis, pneumonia, sinusitis, stomach and intestinal problems, bladder infections, prostate infections, gallbladder infections, rheumatism, gout, impotence and anorgasmia; stimulates adrenals.

Skin and hair: Treats foot odor.

Hints: Recommended oil for sauna, steam bath, and air freshener.

Frankincense

Latin name: Boswellia thuriferia
Obtained from: The resin of the tree
Scent: Balsamic, woody, aromatic, lemonlike
Properties: Benefits skin; acts as uterine tonic, astringent, antiseptic, nerve sedative, diuretic; aids digestion; heals wounds; aids in the formation of scar tissue; eases grippy pains; expels gas; rejuvenates cells and skin; stimulates; acts as anti-inflammatory agent.
General uses: Treats bronchitis, coughs, colds, digestive problems, infections of urinary tract, bladder, and kidneys; treats uterus disorders, excessive menstrual flow, vaginal discharge, gonorrhea, nervousness.
Skin and hair: Helps with general skin care; acts as skin tonic; treats skin inflammation, wounds, cuts, sores, wrinkles; rejuvenates cells.
Emotions and mind: Treats anxiety, restlessness, agitation, worries; recommended oil for meditation; slightly aphrodisiac scent.
Hints: Contraindicated during pregnancy.

Galbanum

Latin name: Ferula galbanifera
Obtained from: The resin of the roots of a plant
Scent: Spicy, woody, balsamic, green
Properties: Acts as nerve sedative; heals wounds; benefits skin.
General uses: Treats uterus weakness, stress, nervousness.

Skin and hair: Treats acne, blemished skin, boils, abscesses, wounds.

Emotions and mind: Treats hysteria, stress, anger, agitation, rage, PMS; recommended oil for meditation blends.

Garlic

Latin name: Allium sativum
Obtained from: The nodule of the plant
Scent: Typically garlic, very pungent
Properties: Acts as antiseptic, bactericide, germicide, fungicide; detoxifies; cleanses blood; relieves spasms; aids digestion; reduces blood pressure; acts as heart tonic; cleanses intestines; stimulates appetite; reduces cholesterol; benefits skin.

General uses: Treats general weakness of the body, infections, colds, bronchitis, asthma, digestive disorders, flatulence, appetite loss, intestinal worms, heart insufficiency, urinary stones, bladder infections, high cholesterol, rheumatism, gout, arthritis, gonorrhea, cancer, AIDS; acts as urine tonic.

Skin and hair: Treats warts, calluses, cold abscesses, scabies, insect bites, skin sores, skin ulcers, corns, fungal infections.

Geranium

Latin name: Pelargonium odorantissimum
Obtained from: The whole plant
Scent: Light, flowery, roselike
Properties: Acts as nerve tonic, nerve sedative; benefits skin; relieves pain; acts as antidepressant, astringent, diuretic; arrests bleeding; heals wounds; aids

in the formation of scar tissue; acts as body tonic, antiseptic, insect repellent, anti-inflammatory agent.

General uses: Treats diabetes, diarrhea, inflammation of the mucous membrane in stomach and intestines, kidney stones, internal ulcers, gastralgia, hemorrhages, jaundice, facial neuralgia, sore throats, uterine cancer, inflammation of mouth (tongue and mucous membrane), hormone imbalance (menopause), pregnancy disorders.

Skin and hair: Helps with general skin care; treats oily skin, skin ulcers, dry eczema, wounds, cuts, sores, skin inflammation, dermatitis, burns; acts as tonic for weak tissue.

Emotions and mind: Treats depression, anxiety; scent makes one feel at harmony.

Hints: Valuable oil for body, massage, and bath oils; provokes possible allergic reactions; acts as insect repellent.

Ginger

Latin name: Zingiber officinale
Obtained from: The root of the plant
Scent: Warm, aromatic, woody
Properties: Acts as antiseptic, stimulant, aphrodisiac; relieves spasms; removes mucus from respiratory tract; acts as stomach tonic; reduces fever; stimulates appetite.
General uses: Treats colds, flu, throat inflammation, angina, fever, headaches, stomach cramps, diarrhea, flatulence, digestive problems, loss of

appetite, sore and tired muscles, arthritis, rheumatism, fatigue, impotence.

Skin and hair: Stimulates skin metabolism.

Emotions and mind: Treats mental confusion.

Hints: Acts as antioxidant and preservative for food and cosmetics.

Grapefruit

Latin name: Citrus maxima

Obtained from: The peel of the fruit

Scent: Light, fresh, fruity, slightly bitter

Properties: Acts as nerve sedative, antiseptic, bactericide, antidepressant, tanning agent; stimulates appetite.

General uses: Treats gall insufficiency, bladder diseases, appetite loss.

Skin and hair: Treats herpes, lifeless skin; stimulates skin metabolism.

Emotions and mind: Treats depression, anxiety, negativity, PMS.

Hints: Freshens air; eliminates cooking odors; acts as antioxidant and preservative for cosmetics.

Hyssop

Latin name: Hyssopus officinalis

Obtained from: The whole plant or bush

Scent: Fresh, aromatic, spicy

Properties: Acts as lung and heart tonic; removes mucus from respiratory tract; stimulates body, mind; balances arterial blood pressure; acts as nerve tonic, antiseptic; relieves spasms, reduces fever; acts as stomach tonic, diuretic, blood cleanser;

stimulates menstrual flow; acts as abortive agent; benefits skin; heals wounds; acts as anti-inflammatory agent.

General uses: Treats asthma, coughs, bronchitis (acute and chronic), flu, colds, whooping cough, abnormally shallow breathing, tuberculosis, high and low blood pressure, physical weakness, inflammation of mouth, throat, and ears; helps with regeneration after illness; treats fever, digestive problems, intestinal worms, flatulence, appetite loss, vaginal discharge, absence of or scanty menstrual flow.

Skin and hair: Treats bruises, skin inflammation, wounds, herpes, eczema, pimples.

Emotions and mind: Treats mental exhaustion and confusion, extreme emotions, loss of concentration.

Hints: Contraindicated during pregnancy. Recommended as an air freshener; helps with infectious diseases. Not to be used if you have epilepsy.

Immortelle

Latin name: Helichrysum angustifolium, gynmocephalum

Obtained from: The whole, blossoming herb

Scent: Tea rose, honeylike, herbal, warm

Properties: Acts as anti-inflammatory agent, fungicide, antiseptic, antiviral agent, diuretic, antiallergic agent; relieves spasms; benefits skin; cleanses blood; acts as liver, gall, and pancreas tonic, lymph stimulant; removes mucus from respiratory tract; acts as tissue tonic.

General uses: Treats migraines, colds, bronchitis, infections of stomach and intestines, throat infections, gall infections, liver weakness, diabetes, sinusitis, menstrual cramps.

Skin and hair: Treats skin inflammations, chronic skin diseases, allergic skin diseases, eczema, psoriasis, acne, blemished skin, burns, viral and bacterial skin diseases; soothes and softens skin; benefits skin after exposure to sun.

Jasmine

Latin name: Jasminus officinale, grandiflorium
Obtained from: The flowers of the bush
Scent: Strong, flowery, honeylike
Properties: Acts as antidepressant, aphrodisiac, uterus tonic, nerve sedative, antiseptic; relieves spasms; increases flow of mother's milk; benefits skin; stimulates uterine contractions.
General uses: Treats coughs, uterus disorders, headaches, absence of or scanty menstrual flow, menstrual cramps; aids in the birth process; treats sore muscles and joints, backaches, impotence and anorgasmia, nervousness.
Skin and hair: Treats dry, sensitive, and inflamed skin, dermatitis, eczema, emotional skin disorders.
Emotions and mind: Treats depression, anxiety, phobia, nervous fatigue, apathy, lack of self-esteem, PMS; scent stimulates inspiration.
Hints: Important oil for women generally and during childbirth. One of the most expensive and exclusive oils but very powerful. Do not take internally as it contains mostly residues of solvents (jasmine is an absolute oil).

Juniper

Latin name: *Juniperus communis*

Obtained from: The dried, ripe berries of the tree

Scent: Fruity, strong, herblike

Properties: Acts as diuretic, body and nerve tonic, bladder and urinary tract tonic, antiseptic, antitoxic agent; relieves spasms; eases grippy pains; expels gas; stimulates body and nerves; stimulates menstrual flow; aids digestion; cleanses blood; acts as stomach tonic; heals wounds; aids in the formation of scar tissue; induces perspiration; acts as aphrodisiac, abortive agent; benefits skin.

General uses: Treats throat infections, coughs, digestive troubles, constipation, flatulence, colic, kidney stones, albuminuria, arteriosclerosis, cirrhosis, urinary tract infections, vaginal discharge, gout, rheumatism, arthritis, intestinal worms, hemorrhoids, dyspepsia, absence of or scanty menstrual flow, menstrual cramps, cystitis, physical weakness, insufficient erection, nervousness, nerve disorders, sore muscles; detoxifies blood.

Skin and hair: Acts as skin cleanser; treats acne, blemished skin, dermatitis, wet eczema, skin ulcers, wounds, cuts, sores, burns, skin infections, cellulite, varicose veins.

Emotions and mind: Treats grief, worry, anxiety, psychic exhaustion and weakness, lack of centeredness.

Hints: Contraindicated during pregnancy. Do not take in large amounts internally.

Lavender

Latin name: *Lavendula, officinalis, vera, angustifolia*
Obtained from: The flowers and stalks of the plant
Scent: Fresh, herblike, balsamic
Properties: Acts as nerve sedative, antidepressant, heart regulator and tonic; benefits skin; stimulates skin and cell rejuvenation; acts as antitoxic agent, antiseptic, diuretic, anticonvulsive; relieves pain, spasms; eases grippy pains; expels gas; stimulates bile flow; acts as deodorant; reduces blood pressure; acts as nerve tonic, spleen tonic; stimulates menstrual flow; heals wounds; acts as anti-inflammatory agent.

General uses: Treats conjunctivitis, eye infections, headaches, migraines, earaches, asthma, bronchitis, tuberculosis, throat infections, whooping cough, flu, fever rash, nerve inflammation, cystitis, inflammation of mucous membranes, colic, diarrhea, diphtheria, dyspepsia, epilepsy, fistula, flatulence, vomiting, gonorrhea, vaginal discharge, pus, sunstroke, high blood pressure, influenza, nervous exhaustion and tension (stress, neurasthenia), fainting, toxification of food, rheumatism, gall disorders, gallstones, heart palpitations, wounds.

Skin and hair: Helps with general skin care; treats dry skin, congested skin, herpes, carbuncles, burns, boils, dermatitis, eczema, skin abscesses, acne, blemished skin, pimples, alopecia, skin ulcers, skin and scalp itching, scabies, skin inflammation, psoriasis, athlete's foot, hair loss, dandruff, body and foot odor; rejuvenates skin; acts as skin tonic.

Emotions and mind: Treats depression, stress, agitation, restlessness, insomnia, anger, severe mood changes; scent gives feeling of space.

Hints: Has mild effects. Recommended oil for children. Acts as pleasant air freshener. There are many different qualities and scents available; look for the more expensive oil. Can be applied full strength on pimples. Very effective in healing burns, scratches, wounds, and sores.

Lemon

Latin name: Citrus limonum, medica

Obtained from: The peel of the fruit

Scent: Typically lemon, light, fresh

Properties: Acts as antiseptic, heart stimulant; increases white blood cells; stimulates immune system; reduces fever; acts as diuretic; arrests bleeding; neutralizes acid; benefits skin; acts as tanning agent; acts as stomach tonic.

General uses: Treats general physical weakness, infections, headaches, migraines, sinusitis, fever, flu, asthma, sore throats, digestion troubles, acidic stomach, vomiting, diarrhea, intestinal disorders, intestinal worms, appetite loss, weak heart, immune system insufficiency, liver insufficiency, rheumatism, gout, arthritis, gonorrhea, syphilis, lack of blood.

Skin and hair: Treats oily skin, congested skin, broken veins, freckles, brittle nails, insect bites; acts as skin cleanser; stimulates excretion from skin of toxins and wastes; helps with hair care for blond hair, coloring blond hair; treats dandruff; helps after exertion in sports.

Emotions and mind: Treats mental fatigue and confusion, lethargy.

Hints: Acts as excellent air freshener; eliminates cooking odors, smoke. Acts as insect repellent. Acts as preventive against infectious diseases when used in aroma lamp. Irritates sensitive skin if high doses are used in bath oil, body oil, or facial oil. Definitely irritates sensitive skin if used in body oil while sunbathing. Long-term internal use not recommended.

Lemongrass
Latin name: Cymbopogon flexousus, citratus
Obtained from: The grass
Scent: Strongly lemonlike
Properties: Acts as antiseptic, diuretic, lymph tonic, deodorant; aids digestion; benefits skin; stimulates body and mind.
General uses: Treats digestive disorders, flatulence, intestinal infection, bladder and kidney diseases, lymph congestion, edema, colds, flu, headaches, rheumatism.
Skin and hair: Treats oily skin, large pores; acts as astringent.
Emotions and mind: Treats loss of concentration, mental fatigue; refreshes the mind.
Hints: May irritate sensitive skin if high doses are used in bath oil, body oil, or facial oil.

Marjoram
Latin name: Origanum majorana

Obtained from: The blossoming twigs of the herb
Scent: Herblike, warm, typically marjoram
Properties: Acts as nerve sedative and tonic; relieves spasms; warms; aids digestion; stimulates menstrual flow, bowel evacuation; reduces sexual desire (anaphrodisiac); acts as antiseptic; eases grippy pains; expels gas; acts as heart tonic; removes mucus from respiratory tract; reduces blood pressure; heals wounds; acts as abortive agent; expands blood vessels.
General uses: Treats colds, asthma, headaches, migraines, dyspepsia, digestive troubles, flatulence, constipation, colic, menstrual cramps, PMS, high blood pressure, vaginal discharge, nervous tension, exhaustion, and tics; treats muscle cramps and tension.
Skin and hair: Treats wounds, cuts, burns, sores.
Emotions and mind: Treats anxiety, grief, sorrow, psychic instability, insomnia, restlessness, agitation, hysteria.
Hints: Contraindicated during pregnancy. Has warming effect in bath oil.

Melissa (Balm, Lemon Balm)
Latin name: Melissa officinalis
Obtained from: The whole herb
Scent: Fresh, lemonlike, strong
Properties: Acts as mind stimulant, antiviral agent, nerve tonic, stomach tonic, uterine tonic, antidepressant, nerve sedative; reduces fever; raises blood pressure; relieves spasms; aids digestion; expels intestinal worms; benefits skin.

General uses: Treats headaches, migraines, colds, fevers, nausea, asthma, allergies, herpes, flatulence, vomiting, stomach and intestinal cramps, diarrhea, intestinal worms, instability of circulation, palpitations, menopausal problems, menstrual problems, uterus disorders, sterility (in women), nervous tension, low blood pressure.

Skin and hair: Treats insect bites, herpes, oily skin, pimples, bruises, eczema, bleeding.

Emotions and mind: Treats insomnia, nightmares, depression, stress, anger, rage, shock, panic, grief, negativity, lethargy, mental fatigue.

Hints: May irritate skin if high doses are used in bath oil, body oil, or facial oil. Provides cooling effect with bath oils and compresses for fever. Acts as insect repellent.

Mimosa

Latin name: Acacia decurrens var. dealbata
Obtained from: The petals of the flower
Scent: Warm, light, bananalike, flowery
Properties: Benefits skin; cleanses blood; acts as liver and gall tonic, anti-inflammatory agent.
General uses: Treats blood toxification, liver and gall insuffiency.
Skin and hair: Helps with general skin care; nourishes skin; acts as humectant; treats skin inflammation.
Hints: This is an expensive absolute oil. It should never be taken internally.

Myrrh

Latin name: Commiphora myrrha, Baslamodendron myrrha

Obtained from: The gum of the tree

Scent: Balsamic, spicy, warm

Properties: Heals wounds; removes mucus from respiratory tract; acts as lung tonic and stimulant, uterine tonic, antiseptic, anti-inflammatory agent, astringent; aids digestion; stimulates menstrual flow; acts as nerve sedative, stomach tonic; benefits skin; acts as abortive agent.

General uses: Treats mouth ulcers and thrush, inflammation of mucous membrane of mouth, colds, coughs, bronchitis, tuberculosis, hoarseness, digestive problems, flatulence, diarrhea, appetite loss, absence of or scanty menstrual flow, hemorrhoids, vaginal discharge, pyorrhea.

Skin and hair: Treats aging skin, wrinkles, wounds, cuts, sores, burns, skin ulcers, fungal skin infections; cools hot skin.

Emotions and mind: Treats agitation, restlessness, emotional overreaction.

Hints: Contraindicated during pregnancy. Myrrh is part of Eastern incense blends for meditation and centering.

Myrtle (African Red, French Green)

Latin name: Myrtus communis

Obtained from: The blossoming twigs of the bush

Scent: Fresh, light, like eucalyptus and sage

Properties: Acts as antiseptic, bactericide, tissue tonic, lung tonic; heals wounds; benefits skin.

General uses: Treats infections of ears, stomach, bladder, and intestines; treats sinusitis, colds, flu, bronchitis, asthma, whooping cough.

Skin and hair: Treats burns, wounds, cuts, skin ulcers, fistulas.

Hints: Recommended for cleansing and disinfecting air if infectious diseases are present.

Neroli (Orange Blossom)

Latin name: Citrus auranthium, bigardia
Obtained from: The blossoms of the tree
Scent: Sweet, spicy-bitter, strong
Properties: Acts as nerve sedative, antidepressant, heart tonic, aphrodisiac, antiseptic, deodorant; benefits skin; aids digestion; relieves spasms; stimulates cell and skin rejuvenation.
General uses: Treats palpitations, chronic diarrhea, nervous tension, impotence and anorgasmia.
Skin and hair: Helps with skin care of all types; treats aging, dry skin, broken veins, redness and irritation of skin; rejuvenates skin.
Emotions and mind: Treats depression, anxiety, grief, anger, hysteria, panic, shock, insomnia, PMS.
Hints: This is an expensive oil, but very effective in treating emotions. Notable oil for rejuvenation of skin and use in floral perfumes and flower waters. Totally nonirritating.

Niaouli

Latin name: Melaleuca viridiflora
Obtained from: The leaves of the tree
Scent: Fresh, like eucalyptus
Properties: Acts as antiseptic, bactericide, tissue tonic; removes mucus from respiratory tract; acts as anti-inflammatory agent; expels intestinal worms.

General uses: Treats all infections, especially of the respiratory system and urinary tract; treats colds, flu, bronchitis, coughs, rheumatism.
Skin and hair: Cleanses skin and wounds; heals wounds; treats acne, blemished skin, boils, burns.
Emotions and mind: Treats mental confusion, lethargy, fatigue.

Nutmeg

Latin name: Myristica fragans
Obtained from: The fruit (nut) of the tree
Scent: Light, spicy
Properties: Acts as body and mind tonic, antiseptic; aids digestion; warms; acts as abortive agent.
General uses: Treats rheumatism, flatulence, digestive problems, absence of or scanty menstrual flow, slow metabolism.
Emotions and mind: Treats mental confusion, fatigue and lethargy.
Hints: Toxic if taken internally in high doses. Not recommended for long-term use. Contraindicated during pregnancy.

Onion

Latin name: Allium cepa
Obtained from: The nodule of the plant
Scent: Pungent, very strong
Properties: Acts as body tonic and stimulant, antiseptic, bactericide, diuretic, hypoglycemic, nerve tonic; removes mucus from respiratory system; benefits skin.
General uses: Treats general physical weakness, me-

tabolism insufficiency, water retention, infections of the respiratory system, flu, migraines, digestive troubles, intestinal worms, diarrhea, irritation of function of glands (swollen lymph glands or nodes), infections of urogenital tract, arteriosclerosis, prostate disorders, diabetes, rheumatism, arthritis, gallstones, general signs of aging.

Skin and hair: Treats inflammation of skin, abscesses, boils, warts, freckles, insect bites.

Emotions and mind: Treats mental fatigue.

Orange

Latin name: Citrus aurantium
Obtained from: The peel of the fruit
Scent: Fresh, light, fruity
Properties: Aids digestion; acts as gall, bladder, and kidney tonic; acts as antidepressant, nerve sedative, disinfectant, heart tonic; reduces fever; relieves spasms; benefits skin; acts as tanning agent.

General uses: Treats digestive problems, flatulence, stomach and intestinal cramps, gall congestion, heart flutter, bladder and kidney ailments, fever, inflammation of the gums, nervousness.

Skin and hair: Helps with general skin care, dry and inflamed skin, cracked skin, calluses, slow skin metabolism, congested skin, cellulite.

Emotions and mind: Treats depression, anxiety, sadness, PMS; scent expands, harmonizes, and brings joy.

Hints: Recommended oil for children because of its mild effects. Works well as an air freshener for kitchen odors.

Oregano

Latin name: Origanum vulgare
Obtained from: The whole blossoming herb
Scent: Spicy, strong, sharp
Properties: Acts as antiseptic, bactericide, virucide, stomach tonic; aids digestion; relieves spasms, stimulates menstrual flow, appetite; acts as abortive agent.
General uses: Treats circulatory disturbances, all internal infections, asthma, tuberculosis, whooping cough, bronchitis, coughs, digestive problems, flatulence, intestinal putrefaction, absence of or scanty menstrual flow, appetite loss, rheumatism.
Skin and hair: Treats cellulite, scabies.
Hints: Toxic in high doses. Contraindicated during pregnancy. May irritate skin if high doses are used in bath oil, body oil, or facial oil. Irritation of mucous membrane if high doses are taken internally. For internal use, substitute the oil of marjoram, which has milder effects.

Parsley

Latin name: Petroselinum crispum
Obtained from: The seed of the herb
Scent: Strong, sharp
Properties: Acts as body stimulant, diuretic, liver, spleen, and uterus tonic; stimulates bowel evacuation.
General uses: Treats ailments of liver, spleen, uterus, urinary tract, gallbladder; treats gallstones, gonorrhea, syphilis, cancer.
Skin and hair: Treats bruises, broken veins.

Patchouli

Latin name: Pogostemon patchouli

Obtained from: The dried and fermented leaves of the herb

Scent: Woody, earthy, erogenous, smoky

Properties: Acts as nerve sedative, antidepressant, aphrodisiac, antiseptic, tonic, deodorant; benefits skin; expels intestinal worms; stimulates cell and skin rejuvenation; heals wounds.

General uses: Treats headaches, colds, fatigue, stomachaches, impotence and anorgasmia, fungal infections of vagina or mouth.

Skin and hair: Helps with general skin care; treats aging skin, wrinkles, wounds.

Emotions and mind: Treats depression, anxiety, self-doubts, restlessness.

Hints: The most popular Asian moth repellent. Basic ingredient of many erogenous perfumes.

Pennyroyal

Latin name: Mentha pulegium

Obtained from: The whole herb

Scent: Like peppermint, slightly bitter

Properties: Acts as nerve tonic, uterine tonic, antiseptic; stimulates body, menstrual flow; relieves spasms; eases grippy pains; expels gas; stimulates and increases bile secretion; aids digestion; removes mucus from respiratory system; reduces fever; acts as stomach tonic, abortive agent.

General uses: Treats asthma, bronchitis, coughs, colds, fevers, headaches, toothaches, mouth sores and ulcers, flatulence, dyspepsia, gastralgia, gallstones, spasms, jaundice, vaginal discharge, menstrual cramps, absence of or scanty menstrual flow, neuralgia, nervous exhaustion (neurasthenia), edema.

Skin and hair: Treats skin itching, insect bites, skin inflammation and irritation.

Emotions and mind: Treats loss of concentration, mental confusion.

Hints: Contraindicated during pregnancy.

Pepper, Black
Latin name: Piper nigrum
Obtained from: The fruit of the seed
Scent: Sharp, spicy, typically pepper
Properties: Aids digestion; warms; acts as stomach tonic, antiseptic, diuretic; eases grippy pains; expels gas; reduces fever; stimulates bowel evacuation; stimulates body, appetite; acts as antitoxin, aphrodisiac, body tonic; relieves pain, spasms.

General uses: Treats colds, flu, coughs, fevers, sore throats, digestive problems, flatulence, intestinal putrefaction, cholera, constipation, vomiting, diarrhea, nausea, heartburn, vertigo, loss of appetite, food toxification, muscle aches, rheumatism, freezing, impotence and anorgasmia.

Hints: May irritate skin if high doses are used in bath oil, body oil, or facial oil. Has a warming effect in bath oil (use as winter bath or to treat colds or rheumatism). Recommended ingredient for an after-sport oil.

Peppermint
Latin name: Mentha piperita, Mentha arvenis, Men tha aquatica

Obtained from: The whole herb

Scent: Fresh, strong, minty

Properties: Relieves pain; reduces fever; acts as anti-septic, stomach tonic; removes mucus from respiratory tract; aids digestion; stimulates bile flow; acts as astringent, liver tonic, nerve tonic, heart tonic; stimulates mind, menstrual flow; promotes constriction of capillaries; eases grippy pains; expels gas; induces perspiration; acts as lymph tonic; expels intestinal worms; benefits skin; acts as anti-inflammatory agent, insect repellent.

General uses: Treats asthma, bronchitis, sinusitis, colds, tuberculosis, fevers, headaches, migraines, toothaches, digestive problems, dyspepsia, flatulence, gastralgia, influenza, nausea, vomiting, diarrhea, cholera, palpitations, neuralgia, galltones, gall constipation, liver ailments, colic, lymph constipation, aches of muscles and joints, menstrual cramps, pruritus (itching) of vagina, vertigo, ringworm, nervous ailments, travel disorders.

Skin and hair: Cleanses skin; treats congested, blemished, and tired facial skin and scalp; treats acne, inflamed skin, scabies, bad breath, insect bites; acts as skin tonic, refreshing hair rinse.

Emotions and mind: Treats shock, fainting, hysteria, mental fatigue, loss of concentration.

Hints: May irritate skin if high doses are used in bath oil, body oil, or facial oil. Has cooling effect in bath. Acts as insect and pest repellent (blend with eucalyptus to repel mice and rats).

Petitgrain

Latin name: Petit Grain bigarade, Citrus bigarade
Obtained from: The leaves, twigs, and unripe fruits
of the tree
Scent: Fresh, flowery, nerolilike
Properties: Acts as nerve tonic, antidepressant; stimulates mind; benefits skin.
General uses: Treats nervous disorders (tension, stomach disorders, nervousness).
Skin and hair: Cleanses skin; acts as skin tonic.
Emotions and mind: Treats mental fatigue, grief, disappointment; has relaxing, harmonizing effect.
Hints: May irritate the skin if used in body oil or facial oil when sunbathing. Has similar scent to neroli but is less expensive.

Pine, Mountain

Latin name: Pinus montana, mugho, pumilio
Obtained from: The needles and twigs of the tree
Scent: Fresh, strong pine scent
Properties: Acts as antiseptic, germicide, anti-inflammatory agent; removes mucus from respiratory system; acts as lung tonic, deodorant.
General uses: Treats colds, bronchitis, weakened immune system, rheumatism, arthritis, gout.
Skin and hair: Treats foot odor.
Hints: Recommended oil for sauna. Acts as good air freshener and air disinfectant if infectious diseases are present.

Pine, Stone

Latin name: Pinus cembra

Obtained from: The branches of the tree

Scent: Balsamic, woody, clear

Properties: Acts as antiseptic; removes mucus from respiratory system; stimulates circulatory system.

General uses: Treats colds, flu, sinusitis, bronchitis, pneumonia, tuberculosis, smoker's cough, rheumatism, muscle tension; regenerates body.

Emotions and mind: Treats loss of concentration, mental fatigue, emotional weakness, loss of energy, nervous depression, anxiety.

Hints: Recommended for sauna and inhalation. Acts as good air freshener and air disinfectant if infec tious diseases are present.

Rose

Latin name: Rosa damascena, Rosa centifolia, Rosa gallica

Obtained from: The petals of the flower

Scent: Flowery, sweet; differs with each kind of rose.

Properties: Acts as antidepressant, heart, liver, uterus, and stomach tonic; acts as aphrodisiac, anti-inflammatory agent, astringent; arrests bleeding; stimulates bowel evacuation; acts as nerve sedative, spleen tonic, stomach tonic; stimulates menstrual flow, cell and skin rejuvenation; heals wounds.

General uses: Treats headaches, nausea, vomiting, constipation, inflammation of gallbladder, uterus disorders, sterility (in women), nervous heart disorders, conjunctivitis, inflammation of the eye, excessive menstrual flow, vaginal discharge, irregular menstruation, nervous tension, insomnia, genital herpes, inflammation of the gums, liver constipation, impotence and anorgasmia.

Skin and hair: Helps with general skin care, baby skin care; acts as skin astringent, skin tonic; treats eczema, wounds, cuts, bruises, dry and inflamed skin, skin allergies.

Emotions and mind: Treats depression, sadness, disappointment, discouragement, grief, PMS.

Hints: This expensive absolute oil should not be taken internally. As an alternative, use rose water, the hydrosol of rose; its effects are similar but harmless, and it is less expensive.

Rosemary

Latin name: Rosemarinus officinalis
Obtained from: The whole blossoming herb
Scent: Woody, strong camphorlike
Properties: Acts as nerve tonic; stimulates nerves, mind; warms; relieves pain, spasms; raises blood pressure; acts as heart tonic, liver tonic, antiseptic, astringent; eases grippy pains; expels gas; stimulates bile flow to intestines; increases bile secretion; aids in digestion; acts as diuretic; stimulates menstrual flow; heals wounds; promotes the formation of scar tissue; benefits skin and hair; acts as abortive agent.

General uses: Treats liver disorders (cirrhosis, jaundice), gallstones, gallbladder inflammation, flu, colds, asthma, colitis, sore muscles, arteriosclerosis, high cholesterol, low blood pressure, diarrhea, influenza, dyspepsia, flatulence, headaches, migraines, palpitations, vaginal discharge, menstrual cramps, pediculosis, rheumatism, gout, nervous disorders, fainting.

Skin and hair: Treats oily and blemished skin, hair loss, wounds, scars, bruises, burns, scabies; helps with hair care for dark hair.

Emotions and mind: Treats loss of memory, mental fatigue, apathy.

Hints: Contraindicated during pregnancy. Contraindicated for use in bath, massage, or high-dosage body oil if you have epilepsy.

Rosewood

Latin name: Aniba roseaodora
Obtained from: The bark and wood of the tree
Scent: Warm, woody, rosy
Properties: Acts as nerve tonic and sedative; benefits skin; acts as euphoriant, deodorant.
General uses: Treats headaches, digestive problems, nervous disorders (tiredness, nervousness, stress).
Skin and hair: Treats dry skin, weakness of connective tissue, body odor; softens skin.
Emotions and mind: Treats overexcitement, emotional confusion, depression, PMS, mood swings.
Hints: This oil is a less expensive substitute for rose oil for the use in the aroma lamp. However, it is similar to rose oil only in terms of its effects on the emotions.

Sage

Latin name: Salvia officinalis
Obtained from: The whole dried herb
Scent: Fresh, strong, herblike, spicy

Properties: Acts as body tonic and stimulant; relieves spasms; acts as tonic, antiseptic, stomach tonic astringent; raises blood pressure.

General uses: Treats gum infections, toothaches, infections of mucous membranes of mouth, mouth fistula, mouth thrush, headaches, sore throats, bronchitis, asthma, slow digestion and excretion, brain strokes, menstrual cramps, absence of or scanty menstrual flow, menopausal problems (hot flashes, sweating), low blood pressure.

Skin and hair: Treats oily and blemished skin, eczema, hair loss, insect bites; balances and cleanses skin; acts as astringent.

Emotions and mind: Treats loss of concentration, mental fatigue.

Hints: Never take the oil internally as it can cause cramps and toxification even in small doses. Contraindicated during pregnancy or if you have epilepsy. Acts as strong air disinfectant if infectious diseases are present. As an alternative, use clary sage, which is milder.

Sandalwood

Latin name: Santalum album
Obtained from: The wood of the tree
Scent: Sweet, woody, erogenous, balsamic
Properties: Removes mucus from the respiratory system; acts as antidepressant, nerve sedative, aphrodisiac, antiseptic, diuretic, anti-inflammatory agent, astringent, tonic; eases grippy pains; expels gas; stimulates cell and skin rejuvenation; benefits skin; relieves spasms.

General uses: Treats coughs, inflammation of the mucous membrane, bronchitis, sinusitis, hiccups, tuberculosis, vomiting, heartburn, bladder and uterus disorders, cystitis, prostatitis, gonorrhea, vaginal discharge, laryngitis, vomiting, impotence and anorgasmia, nervous tension, nausea.

Skin and hair: Helps with general skin care; treats dry, blemished, and inflamed skin; treats eczema, itching, acne; rejuvenates skin.

Emotions and mind: Treats stress, anxiety, insomnia, aggression, egoism; has centering and relaxing effect.

Hints: Do not take the oil internally if you have kidney inflammation. The scent of sandalwood is very helpful for meditation and relaxation.

Sassafras

Latin name: Ocotea cymbarum
Obtained from: The bark and roots of the tree
Scent: Spicy, fresh, herblike
Properties: Acts as body tonic, anti-inflammatory agent; induces perspiration; stimulates body, menstrual flow.
General uses: Treats general physical weakness, flatulence, rheumatism, gout, absence of or scanty menstrual flow, syphilis, fever; regenerates body.
Skin and hair: Treats skin inflammation and infection.
Hints: Contraindicated during pregnancy. May irritate skin if high doses are used in bath oil, body oil, or facial oil.

Savory

Latin name: Satureja montana

Obtained from: The whole plant
Scent: Fresh, herblike, medicinal, thymelike
Properties: Aids in digestion, acts as strong antiseptic, stomach tonic, aphrodisiac; removes mucus from respiratory system; relieves spasms; expels intestinal worms; heals wounds.
General uses: Treats digestive problems, flatulence, diarrhea, weak or nervous stomach, intestinal cramps, intestinal worms, impotence and anorgasmia.
Skin and hair: Treats insect bites, wounds.

Tangerine
Latin name: Citrus madurensis
Obtained from: The peel of the fruit
Scent: Fresh, fruity, sweet
Properties: Acts as nerve sedative, stomach tonic, relieves pain, spasms; stimulates appetite, stomach, intestines, gall.
General uses: Treats digestive problems, weakened liver and stomach, loss of appetite, sore muscles, nervousness.
Emotions and mind: Treats anxiety, emotional tension, grief, sadness, insomnia, PMS.

Tarragon
Latin name: Artemisia dracunulus
Obtained from: The whole herb
Scent: Strong, spicy, celery and aniselike
Properties: Acts as stomach tonic; aids digestion; relieves spasms; stimulates appetite, menstrual flow; acts as antiseptic, abortive agent.

General uses: Treats loss of appetite, digestive problems, flatulence, hiccups, intestinal worms, general weakness of the body, rheumatism, absence of or scanty menstrual flow.

Hints: Contraindicated during pregnancy.

Tea Tree

Latin name: Melaleuca alternifolia
Obtained from: The leaves of the tree
Scent: Fresh, medical, strong, sharp
Properties: Acts as fungicide, bactericide, germicide; expels intestinal worms; benefits skin; heals wounds.
General uses: Treats all infections, internal and external (of vagina, intestines, skin, athlete's foot, etc.); treats inflammation of mucous membrane of the mouth, weakened immune system.
Skin and hair: Treats acne, blemished skin, pimples, fungal skin infections, hair loss, wounds, cuts, burns; stimulates scalp.
Hints: Tea tree oil is totally nontoxic.

Thyme

Latin name: Thymus vulgaris
Obtained from: The blossoming twigs of the herb
Scent: Strong, medical, sweet
Properties: Acts as antiseptic, bactericide, fungicide, nerve tonic; relieves spasms; removes mucus from respiratory system; stimulates body, mind; acts as diuretic; induces perspiration; raises blood pressure; stimulates menstrual flow; heals wounds; acts as wound disinfectant, abortive agent.

General uses: Treats colds, flu, bronchitis, sinusitis, inflammation of the mucous membrane, whooping cough, tuberculosis, asthma, sore throats, fungal infections, circulatory irritations, infections of urinary tract, intestinal worms, rheumatism, gout, arthritis, vaginal discharge, absence of or scanty menstrual flow, lack of white blood cells, weakened immune system, low blood pressure; helps body regenerate after illness.

Skin and hair: Helps with mouth and gum care; treats wounds, cuts, burns, bruises, boils, scabies, lice, athlete's foot.

Emotions and mind: Treats mental fatigue, general weakness, loss of concentration, lethargy; stimulates intelligence.

Hints: There are two essential oils of thyme: a white one with mild effects and a red one with strong effects. Both are contraindicated during pregnancy or if you have epilepsy or an overfunction of the thyroid gland. This oil should never be applied undiluted on the skin.

Tuberose

Latin name: Polianthes tuberosa

Obtained from: The flower of the plant

Scent: Very sweet, flowery, and strong

Emotions and mind: Centers and strengthens emotionally; acts as a mild aphrodisiac.

Hints: This very expensive absolute oil is generally used to give creams, lotions, and perfumes a very flowery and sweet scent. Not for internal use.

Tuja

Latin name: Tuja occidentalis

Obtained from: The bark and leaves of the tree

Properties: Removes mucus from respiratory system; acts as diuretic, antiseptic; stimulates body.

General uses: Treats cystitis, prostatitis, rheumatism, intestinal worms, cancer; aids in the prevention of sexually transmitted diseases.

Skin and hair: Treats warts.

Hints: Contraindicated if you have epilepsy. Not for internal use; it can cause cramps. Use low dosages for all applications.

Turpentine

Latin name: Pinus pineaster

Obtained from: The resin of the tree

Scent: Strong, medical, woody, pinelike

Properties: Acts as antiseptic; removes mucus from respiratory system; relieves spasms.

General uses: Treats bronchitis, whooping cough, tuberculosis, infections of the urinary and genital tract, cystitis, intestinal cramps, flatulence, intestinal worms, gallstones, neuralgia, gout, arthritis, rheumatism.

Skin and hair: Treats eczema, lice, scabies, wounds.

Hints: To be used in low doses. High doses can cause irritation of the kidneys.

Verbena

Latin name: Verbena triphylla, Aloisia triphylla

Obtained from: The leaves of the plant

Scent: Slightly lemonlike, light, fresh, sweet

Properties: Acts as body tonic, euphoriant, stomach tonic, antidepressant; stimulates mind.

General uses: Treats colds, flu, loss of appetite, congestion, digestive problems, fainting, insomnia; aids in birthing process.

Skin and hair: Treats oily and blemished skin, acne, weakness of connective tissue; acts as effective oil to use after physical exertion.

Emotions and mind: Treats mental fatigue, loss of concentration, depression, mood swings; motivates and inspires; stimulates and refreshes.

Hints: Stimulates uterine contractions during birth process but contraindicated during pregnancy. Recommended scent for people who work with their minds.

Vetiver

Latin name: Vetivera zizanoides

Obtained from: The roots of the grass

Scent: Earthy, woody, musty

Properties: Acts as nerve sedative and tonic; benefits skin.

General uses: Treats nervousness, nervous disorders (neurasthenia), stress.

Skin and hair: Treats mature, dry, and irritated skin; regenerates skin; strengthens connective tissue (during pregnancy); stimulates bust growth.

Emotions and mind: Treats sense of rootlessness.

Violet, Blue

Latin name: Viola odorata

Obtained from: The flower and leaves of the plant

Scent: Herblike, pepperlike, like fall foliage

Properties: Acts as nerve tonic and sedative; aids digestion; acts as respiratory tonic, anti-inflammatory agent.

General uses: Treats headaches, colds, coughs, whooping cough, throat infections, bronchitis, flatulence, constipation, internal ulcers, cancer, nervousness, stress.

Skin and hair: Treats skin inflammation.

Emotions and mind: Treats annoyance, overexcitement, restlessness.

Hints: This is an absolute oil; not to be taken internally.

Ylang-Ylang

Latin name: Cananga odorata

Obtained from: The flowers of the tree

Scent: Strong, sweet, erogenous, flowery

Properties: Acts as antidepressant, aphrodisiac; reduces blood pressure; lowers adrenaline; benefits skin; acts as nerve sedative, antiseptic.

General uses: Treats abnormally fast breathing, high blood pressure, palpitations, insomnia, impotence and anorgasmia, nervous tension, stress, nervous exhaustion.

Skin and hair: Treats oily, aging, dry, or strained skin; stimulates bust growth.

Emotions and mind: Treats anger, rage, anxiety, low self-esteem, nervous depression, PMS, emotional coldness.

Hints: This scent lasts a very long time and is very intense. Use dosages carefully.

18
Index of Symptoms or Effects and Corresponding Essential Oils

Abortive Agents
basil, camphor, carrot, cedarwood, clove, frankincense, hyssop, juniper, marjoram, myrrh, nutmeg, oregano, pennyroyal, peppermint, rosemary, sage, sassafras

Abscess, cold
bergamot, chamomile, garlic, lavender, tea tree

Abscess, warm
onion

Acne
bergamot, cajeput, camphor, cedarwood, chamomile, immortelle, juniper, lavender, lemon, niauoli, peppermint, sandalwood, tea tree

Aging
garlic, lemon, onion, thyme

AIDS
See Immune system, strengthening of.

Air cleansers and refreshers
cinnamon, fir, lemon, orange, peppermint, pine

Air or room disinfectants
bergamot, cinnamon, clove, eucalyptus, juniper, sage,
thyme

Albuminuria (albumin in the urine)
juniper

Alcoholism, detoxification from
fennel

Allergies, general
immortelle, Melissa

Allergies, skin
Melissa, rose

Analgesic
See Pain.

Anaphrodisiac (reducing sexual desire)
marjoram

Anemia
lemon, Roman chamomile, thyme

Angina
bergamot, ginger, lemon, thyme

Anorgasmia
anise, cardamom, cinnamon, coriander, fir, juniper,
pepper, onion, savory (physical); jasmine, sandalwood
(hormonal); clary sage, patchouli, rose, ylang-ylang
(emotional)

Antidepressants
basil, bergamot, camphor, chamomile, clary sage, geranium, grapefruit, jasmine, lavender, neroli, patchouli, rose, sandalwood, verbena, ylang-ylang

Antiseptics
All essential oils inhibit the growth of organisms (bacterias, germs), but some are more effective: bergamot, cajeput, cinnamon, eucalyptus, fir, garlic, immortelle, juniper, lavender, niauoli, onion, pine, rose, rosemary, savory, tea tree, thyme

Antiviral agents (killing viruses)
bergamot, eucalyptus, garlic, Melissa, tea tree, thyme

Anxiety
basil, benzoin, bergamot, clary sage, frankincense, geranium, grapefruit, jasmine, juniper, lavender, marjoram, Melissa, neroli, orange, patchouli, rose, sandalwood, vanilla, verbena, vetiver, ylang-ylang

Apathy
bergamot, cajeput, clary sage, jasmine

Aphrodisiacs (stimulating sex drive)
cardamom, cinnamon, coriander, fir, juniper, pepper, savory (physical); clary sage, frankincense, jasmine, patchouli, rose, sandalwood, ylang-ylang (psychosomatic)

Appetite, increasing
caraway, cardamom, coriander, garlic, ginger, grapefruit, hyssop, lemon, myrrh, oregano, pepper, sage, tangerine, tarragon, vetiver

Appetite, reducing
fennel, lemon, onion (reducing hunger); bergamot, juniper (balancing appetite)

Arterial infection
garlic, lemon, marjoram, onion

Arteriosclerosis
garlic, juniper, lemon, onion, rosemary

Arthritis
See Rheumatism.

Asthma
anise, benzoin, bergamot, cypress, eucalyptus, garlic, hyssop, lavender, lemon, marjoram, Melissa, myrtle, oregano, pennyroyal, peppermint, rosemary, sage, thyme

Astringents
cedarwood, cypress, frankincense, geranium, juniper, lemon, myrrh, patchouli, peppermint, rose, rosemary, sandalwood

Athlete's foot
See Fungicides.

Back pain
See also Lumbago; Pain.
lavender, marjoram, pepper, rosemary

Bactericides
See Antiseptics.

Baldness
birch, clary sage, lavender, rosemary

Bed-wetting
cypress

Birthing (inducing birth; easing pain)
clary sage, jasmine, lavender, pennyroyal

Bladder, infection of
bergamot, cajeput, eucalyptus, fennel, juniper, lavender, myrtle, sandalwood, thyme, tuja

Bladder, inflammation of (cystitis)
bergamot, cedarwood, eucalyptus, juniper, lavender, sandalwood

Bladder, inflammation of mucous membrane of
bergamot, cedarwood, eucalyptus, garlic, juniper, lavender, Roman chamomile, sandalwood

Bladder and painful urination
cedarwood, juniper

Bleeding
See Blood, arresting bleeding of.

Blepharitis (inflammation of the eyelids)
See Eyes, conjunctivis in.

Blisters
eucalyptus

Blood, arresting bleeding of
cypress, geranium, lemon, rose

Blood, cleansing and purifying
eucalyptus, fennel, garlic, juniper, rose

Blood, excessive loss of (menstruation)
cinnamon, cypress, frankincense, pennyroyal, rose

Blood, lack of
lemon, onion, Roman chamomile, thyme

Blood, thinning
lemon

Blood pressure
See Circulation.

Blood sugar, low (hypoglycemia)
eucalyptus

Boils
bergamot, clary sage, lavender, lemon, onion, niauoli,
Roman chamomile, thyme

Boredom and lethargy
cardamom, juniper, lemongrass, rosemary

Brain strokes
sage

Breasts, engorgement of
geranium, peppermint

Breasts, insufficient milk from
fennel, jasmine

Breasts, stimulating growth of
geranium, vetiver, ylang-ylang

Bronchitis
basil, benzoin, blue violet, camphor, cedarwood, cinnamon, eucalyptus, fir, frankincense, garlic, hyssop, immortelle, lemon, pennyroyal, peppermint, rosemary, sage, sandalwood, stony pine, thyme, turpentine

Bruises
parsley, rosemary, sage

Burns
lavender, myrtle, Roman chamomile, rosemary

Calluses
clove, garlic, orange

Cancer, supportive treatment of
See also Immune system.
blue violet, clove, cypress, eucalyptus, garlic, geranium, hyssop, onion, parsley, tea tree, tuja

Carbuncles
bergamot, lavender

Cellulite
cypress, fennel, juniper, lavender, orange, oregano

Cholesterol, high
rosemary

Cholera
camphor, eucalyptus, pepper, peppermint

Circulation, reducing (for hypertension)
clary sage, garlic, lavender, marjoram, Melissa, ylang-ylang

Circulation, stimulating (for hypotension)
camphor, cinnamon, cumin, hyssop, pine, rosemary

Circulation, unbalanced or irritated
cypress, garlic, hyssop, thyme

Cirrhosis
See Liver, inflammation of.

Colds
anise, basil, benzoin, cajeput, camphor, cedarwood, cinnamon, eucalyptus, garlic, ginger, hyssop, immortelle, lavender, marjoram, Melissa, pennyroyal, pepper, peppermint, pine, rosemary, sage, thyme, verbena

Colic
anise, benzoin, camphor, cardamom, clary sage, fennel, hyssop, juniper, lavender, marjoram, Melissa, pepper, peppermint, Roman chamomile

Colitis
bergamot, lavender, neroli, Roman chamomile, ylang-ylang

Conjunctivitis
See Eyes, conjunctivitis in.

Connective tissue, weakness of
rose, rosewood

Constipation
See Intestines, constipation and.

Convalescense
See Regeneration after illness.

Convulsions
clary sage, lavender, neroli, Roman chamomile, rose,
ylang-ylang

Corns
garlic, fennel

Cough
anise, benzoin, cardamom, cinnamon, cypress, eucalyptus, fir, frankincense, hyssop, jasmine, juniper,
marjoram, myrrh, myrtle, niauoli, pennyroyal, pepper, peppermint, rosemary, sandalwood, stone pine,
thyme

Cough, whooping
basil, cypress, hyssop, lavender, myrtle, pennyroyal,
rosemary, thyme, violet

Cramps
basil, bergamot, camphor, cardamom, clary sage, cori-

ander, cypress, eucalyptus, fennel, hyssop, juniper, lavender, marjoram, pennyroyal, pepper, peppermint, Roman chamomile, rose, rosemary, sandalwood

Cystitis
See Urinary tract.

Deodorants
benzoin, bergamot, clary sage, fir (for feet); cypress, eucalyptus, lavender, patchouli, rosewood

Depression
See Antidepressants.

Dermatitis
See Skin care, dermatitis and.

Diabetes
eucalyptus, geranium, juniper, onion

Diarrhea
camphor, clove, cypress, eucalyptus, garlic, geranium, ginger, lavender, Melissa, myrrh, neroli, onion, orange, pepper, peppermint, Roman chamomile, rosemary, sandalwood, savory

Digestive aids
basil, bergamot, cardamom, frankincense, hyssop, marjoram, Melissa, pepper, rosemary

Digestive problems
See Stomach, digestive problems and.

Diphtheria
bergamot, eucalyptus, lavender

Disinfectant
See Air or room disinfectants.

Diuretics
anise, benzoin, camphor, cardamom, eucalyptus, fennel, garlic, geranium, juniper, lavender, onion, pepper, sage

Dizziness
See Fainting.

Dyspepsia
See Stomach, digestive problems and.

Earaches and inflammation of ears (otitis)
basil, blue chamomile, cajeput, lavender, hyssop, myrtle, Roman chamomile

Edema
garlic, geranium, onion, rosemary

Emotional coldness
clary sage, grapefruit, jasmine, orange, patchouli, ylang-ylang

Emotional trauma and fatigue
geranium, grapefruit, neroli, rose

Epilepsy
basil, lavender, rosemary; contraindicated: camphor, hyssop, sage, tuja

Euphoriants
clary sage, grapefruit, jasmine, rose

Eyes, conjunctivitis in
lavender, Roman chamomile, rose

Eyes, fogginess of
rosemary

Eyes, infection of lids of
geranium, lemon, Roman chamomile

Eyes, tired
Lavender, Roman chamomile, rose

Fainting
basil, bergamot, camphor, fir, lavender, Melissa, peppermint, pine, Roman chamomile, rosemary, savory

Fear
See Anxiety.

Fever
basil, bergamot, camphor, eucalyptus, hyssop, lemon, Melissa, pennyroyal, pepper, peppermint, Roman chamomile, sassafras, tea tree

Fistula
lavender, myrrh

Flatulence
anise, bergamot, caraway, cinnamon, clary sage, clove, hyssop, juniper, lavender, lemon, marjoram, myrrh, nutmeg, orange, oregano, pennyroyal, pepper, peppermint, Roman chamomile, rosemary, sandalwood, savory

Fleas
clove, eucalyptus, geranium, lavender, lemon, rosemary

Foot odor
See Deodorants.

Fungicides
angelica, camphor, cinnamon, citronella, fennel, immortelle, myrrh, nutmeg, tea tree, thyme

Gall, stimulating
carrot, grapefruit, lavender, rose, rosemary

Gallbladder, infection or inflammation of
fir, parsley, rose, rosemary

Gallbladder, stimulation of bile flow in
lavender, pennyroyal, peppermint, Roman chamomile, rosemary

Gallstones
bergamot, eucalyptus, lavender, onion, parsley, pennyroyal, peppermint, rosemary, turpentine

Gastralgia
See Stomach, gastralgia or gastritis of.

Gastritis
See Stomach, gastralgia or gastritis of.

Genitals, gonorrhea affecting
benzoin, bergamot, cedarwood, eucalyptus, garlic, frankincense, jasmine, lavender, lemon, parsley, sandalwood

Genitals, itching of (pruritus)
bergamot, clary sage, lavender, Roman chamomile

Genitals, lack of erection affecting
fir, juniper, savory

Genitals, mucus discharge from
bergamot, cedarwood, eucalyptus, geranium, frankincense, juniper, patchouli, lavender, sandalwood

Genitals, syphilis affecting
lemon, parsley, sassafras

Genitals, vaginal discharge from
benzoin, bergamot, clary sage, eucalyptus, frankincense, hyssop, lavender, marjoram, myrrh, pennyroyal, rose, rosemary, sage, sandalwood, tea tree, thyme

Genital herpes
See Herpes.

Germicides
See Antiseptics.

Gout
cajeput, camphor, fir, garlic, juniper, lemon, rosemary, sassafras, thyme, turpentine

Grief
See Antidepressants.

Gums, bleeding of
cypress, myrrh, sage, thyme

Gums, care of
fennel, lemon, myrrh, sage, thyme

Gums, inflammation of
clove, lemon, sage, thyme

Hair, brittle
jojoba

Hair, dandruff from
clary sage, eucalyptus, frankincense, patchouli, rosemary, tea tree

Hair, dry
carrot, frankincense, geranium, lavender

Hair, general care of
cedarwood, chamomile (blond hair only), clary sage, lavender, lemon (blond hair only), patchouli, rosemary, rosewood

Hair, loss of
birch, cajeput, cedarwood, clary sage, lavender, rosemary, sage, thyme

Hair, oily
bergamot, cedarwood, clary sage, cypress, juniper

Hay fever
See Allergies, general.

Headache
eucalyptus, jasmine, lavender (fever headache), lemon, marjoram, Melissa, Roman chamomile, rose, rosemary, sage

Heart, aching
rose

Heart, flutter or palpitations of (sedative)
caraway, lavender, Melissa, neroli, peppermint, Roman chamomile, rose, ylang-ylang

Heartburn
See Stomach, heartburn and.

Heart failure
camphor, cumin, rosemary

Heart stimulant
camphor, cumin, hyssop, rosemary

Heart tonic
cumin, garlic, hyssop, lavender, marjoram, Melissa, neroli, peppermint, rose, rosemary

Hemorrhagia
See Blood, arresting bleeding of.

Hemorrhoids
cypress, frankincense, juniper, myrrh

Herpes
bergamot, camphor, eucalyptus, grapefruit, Melissa, rose, tea tree

Hiccups
basil, caraway, fennel, tarragon

Hoarseness
cypress, jasmine, lemon, myrrh, thyme

Hormones, balancing estrogen
fennel, geranium, sage

Hypertension
See Circulation, reducing.

Hyperventilation
frankincense, ylang-ylang

Hypotension
See Circulation, stimulating.

Hysteria
See Nerves.

Immune system, strengthening of
angelica, cajeput, eucalyptus, garlic, tea tree

Impotence
anise, cardamom, cinnamon, coriander, fir, juniper, pepper, onion, savory (physical); jasmine, sandalwood (hormonal); clary sage, patchouli, rose, ylang-ylang (emotional)

Infections
angelica, cinnamon, clove, fir, garlic, immortelle, lemon, myrtle, niauoli, oregano, tea tree, thyme

Infectious diseases
See Air or room disinfectants.

Inflammation
chamomile, clary sage, eucalyptus, immortelle, lavender, myrrh, peppermint, rose, sandalwood

Insect bites
clove, garlic, lavender, lemon, Melissa, onion, pennyroyal, sage, sassafras, savory

Insect repellents
basil, cedarwood, citronella, clove, cypress, eucalyptus, geranium, lemon, lemongrass, Melissa, onion, pennyroyal, peppermint

Insomnia
See also Nerves.
basil, benzoin, bergamot, camphor, lavender, marjoram, neroli, orange, Roman chamomile, rose, sandalwood, verbena, ylang-ylang

Intestines, colic in
anise, benzoin, bergamot, cardamom, fennel, juniper, lavender, peppermint

Intestines, colon infection of
garlic, immortelle, onion, myrtle, tea tree, thyme

Intestines, constipation and
camphor, basil, fennel, lavender, marjoram, pepper, Roman chamomile, rose

Intestines, infection of
bergamot, garlic, lavender, pepper, Roman chamomile, rosemary

Intestines, putrefaction of
cardamom, cinnamon, coriander, garlic, lemon, marjoram, onion

Intestines, worms in
bergamot, caraway, eucalyptus, hyssop, juniper, lemon, Melissa, onion, peppermint, Roman chamomile, savory, tarragon, thyme, tuja, turpentine

Invigoration
cardamom, coriander, juniper, lemongrass, rosemary

Irritability
benzoin, frankincense, Roman chamomile, rose, ylang-ylang

Itching
See Skin care, itching and.

Kidney, inflammation of
cedarwood, eucalyptus, frankincense, Roman chamomile

Kidney, inflammation of pelvis around
cedarwood, juniper

Kidney, tonic for
cedarwood, clary sage, eucalyptus, juniper, sandalwood

Kidney stones
fennel, geranium, juniper

Laryngitis
benzoin, frankincense, sandalwood

Laxative
caraway, fennel, juniper, marjoram, pepper, rose, sage, tuja, verbena, violet

Lethargy
See Euphoriants; Mind, mental fatigue; Stimulants, body.

Leukocytosis, stimulants for
all oils, especially bergamot, lavender, Roman chamomile

Lice
clove, cinnamon, eucalyptus, geranium, lavender, lemon, lemongrass, oregano, rosemary, thyme, turpentine

Liver, congestion of
cypress, Roman chamomile, rose, rosemary

Liver, detoxifying
juniper

Liver, hepatitis of
rosemary

Liver, inflammation of (cirrhosis)
lemon, juniper, rosemary

Liver, irritation of
cypress, lemon, Roman chamomile, rose, rosemary, sage, thyme

Liver, jaundice of
cypress, geranium, lemon, Roman chamomile, rosemary, thyme

Liver, tonic for
carrot, fennel, lemon, tangerine

Lumbago
See also Back pain.
ginger

Lymphatic system, inflammation of nodes of
juniper, lavender, onion, sage

Lymphatic system, stimulant for
fennel, immortelle, oregano, rosemary, tarragon

Measles
eucalyptus

Menopause, disorders during (hot flashes, sweating)
sage (sweating); cypress, fennel, geranium, Roman chamomile (hormonal balance)

Menstruation, excessive loss of blood (menorrhagia)
cypress, rose

Menstruation, irregular
clary sage, Melissa, rose

Menstruation, painful (menstrual cramps)
anise, benzoin, bergamot, caraway, carrot, clary sage, cypress, ginger, jasmine, marjoram, Melissa, pennyroyal, peppermint, rose, rosemary, tea tree

Menstruation, scanty or late (amenorrhea)
anise, caraway, carrot, cinnamon, clary sage, clove, cypress, fennel, hyssop, jasmine, juniper, lavender,

Melissa, myrrh, nutmeg, oregano, pennyroyal, Roman chamomile, rosemary, sage, sassafras, tarragon

Metabolism, balancing
lemon

Migraine
anise, basil, chamomile, eucalyptus, lavender, lemon, marjoram, Melissa, onion, rosemary

Mind, mental fatigue, loss of concentration, poor memory, and
basil, cardamom, citronella, lemon, lemongrass, peppermint, rosemary, verbena

Mood swings
bergamot, benzoin, clary sage, frankincense, geranium, jasmine, rosewood

Mouth, bad breath in
bergamot, cardamom, eucalyptus, fennel, peppermint, thyme

Mouth, inflammation of
bergamot, hyssop

Mouth, inflammation of mucous membrane of
geranium, lemon, myrrh, sage, tea tree

Mouth, thrush in
geranium, myrrh

Mouth, ulcer on
myrrh, pennyroyal, sage

Muscles, aching or sore
cajeput, ginger, juniper, lavender, lemon, pepper, Roman chamomile, rosemary, tangerine

Muscles, tension or stiffness in
lavender, pepper, tangerine

Muscles, tonic for
See Tonic, body.

Nausea
basil, cardamom, lavender, fennel, Melissa, pepper, peppermint, rose, sandalwood

Nerves, nervous tension, and stress
angelica, basil, benzoin, bergamot, camphor, carrot, cypress, galbanum, geranium, grapefruit, jasmine, lavender, marjoram, Melissa, neroli, patchouli, petitgrain, pine, Roman chamomile, rose, rosewood, sandalwood, tangerine, vetiver, ylang-ylang

Nerves, tonic for
clary sage, cypress, lavender, marjoram, onion, petitgrain, rosemary, sage, thyme

Nerves and nervousness
bergamot, benzoin, camphor, chamomile, lavender, marjoram, myrrh, neroli, orange, Roman chamomile, tangerine

Neuralgia
eucalyptus, geranium, pennyroyal, peppermint, Roman chamomile, turpentine

Neurasthenia (mental fatigue)
clary sage, lavender, marjoram

Nightmares
See Anxiety; Nerves.

Nosebleed
cypress, frankincense, lemon

Obesity
fennel, juniper

Overexcitement
See Nerves.

Oxidation, inhibiting (food, cosmetics)
benzoin, ginger, grapefruit

Pain (analgesics)
bergamot, camphor, eucalyptus, geranium, lavender, marjoram, peppermint, Roman chamomile, rosemary

Paralysis
basil, lavender, peppermint, rosemary, sage

Phobia
See also Anxiety.
jasmine, Melissa, neroli

PMS, moodiness and
bergamot, clary sage, galbanum, geranium, jasmine, neroli, patchouli, rose, rosewood, tangerine ylang-ylang

PMS, water retention and
fennel, geranium, juniper, rosemary

Pneumonia
camphor, fir

Poisoning, food
garlic, lavender, pepper, thyme

Polyps
basil

Prostatitis
fir, jasmine, onion, tuja

Pruritus
See Genitals, itching of.

Psoriasis
See Skin care, psoriasis and.

Regeneration after illness
basil, clary sage, clove, ginseng, hyssop, lemon, rosemary, thyme

Respiratory system, inflammation of mucous membrane of
cajeput, cedarwood, hyssop, lavender, myrrh, sandalwood, stone pine

Respiratory system, removing secretion and mucus from (expectorant)
basil, benzoin, bergamot, cedarwood, eucalyptus, hyssop, marjoram, myrrh, pennyroyal, peppermint, sandalwood

Rheumatism
camphor, citronella, coriander, cypress, eucalyptus, fir, garlic, ginger, juniper, lavender, lemon, lemongrass, marjoram, nutmeg, onion, oregano, pepper, rosemary, sage, sassafras, thyme, tuja, turpentine

Ringworm
bergamot, cinnamon, clove, lavender, peppermint, thyme, turpentine

Scabies
bergamot, lavender, peppermint, rosemary

Scarlet fever
eucalyptus

Sedatives
See Nerves.

Shingles
eucalyptus, geranium, Melissa, peppermint, rose

Shock
camphor, Melissa, peppermint

Sinusitis
cajeput, eucalyptus, fir, garlic, lavender, lemon, peppermint, tea tree, thyme

Skin care, acne and
bergamot, cajeput, camphor, cedarwood, galbanum, geranium, juniper, lavender, myrtle, patchouli, peppermint, Roman chamomile, tea tree

Skin care, astringent oils and
bergamot, cedarwood, cypress, frankincense, geranium, immortelle, juniper, lemon, myrrh, myrtle, orange, rose, rosemary, sandalwood

Skin care, broken veins and
cypress, parsley, Roman chamomile, rose

Skin care, calluses, horn skin and
clove, garlic, orange

Skin care, cleansing oils for
basil, juniper, lemon, niauoli, peppermint

Skin care, congested skin and
basil, juniper, lemon, niauoli, peppermint

Skin care, cracked or chapped skin and
carrot, immortelle, lavender, myrrh, patchouli, rose, sandalwood

Skin care, dermatitis and
cedarwood, hyssop, immortelle, juniper

Skin care, dry skin and
cedarwood, geranium, immortelle, jasmine, lavender, rose, rosewood, sandalwood, ylang-ylang

Skin care, freckles and
lemon, onion

Skin care, infections and
blue chamomile, eucalyptus, garlic, myrrh, Roman chamomile, rosemary

Skin care, inflammation or rush and
benzoin, bergamot, blue chamomile, cedarwood, eucalyptus, hyssop, immortelle, jasmine, lavender, myrrh, niauoli, patchouli, peppermint, Roman chamomile, sandalwood

Skin care, itching and
benzoin, jasmine, lavender, peppermint, Roman chamomile

Skin care, mature skin, rejuvenating oils and
frankincense, lavender, myrrh, neroli, patchouli, rose, sandalwood, vetiver

Skin care, normal skin and
bergamot, jasmine, lavender, neroli, Roman chamomile, rose, rosewood, ylang-ylang

Skin care, oily skin and
bergamot, camphor, cedarwood, cypress, frankincense, geranium, juniper, lavender, lemon, orange, peppermint, rose, rosemary, sandalwood, ylang-ylang

Skin care, pimples, blemished skin and
galbanum, immortelle, lavender, lemon, rosemary sage, tea tree, thyme

Skin care, psoriasis and
bergamot, galbanum, lavender

Skin care, sensitive and irritated skin and
cedarwood, geranium, lemon

Skin care, sensitive skin and
jasmine, neroli, orange, Roman chamomile, rose

Skin care, ulcers and
benzoin, camphor, eucalyptus, garlic, geranium, lavender, onion, rosemary

Skin care, wrinkles and
anise, carrot, cypress, fennel, frankincense, neroli

Spasms (antispasmodics)
basil, bergamot, camphor, cardamom, clary sage, coriander, cypress, eucalyptus, fennel, hyssop, juniper, lavender, marjoram, pennyroyal, pepper, peppermint, Roman chamomile, rose, rosemary

Spleen, tonic for (splenetic)
fennel, parsley, pepper, Roman chamomile, rose

Sprains
camphor, eucalyptus, lavender, rosemary

Sterility (in women)
geranium, rose

Stimulants, body
camphor, cardamom, coriander, eucalyptus, garlic, juniper, lemon, onion, pepper, peppermint, sage, thyme

Stomach, digestive problems and (dyspepsia)
basil, bergamot, cardamom, eucalyptus, fennel, frankincense, juniper, lavender, marjoram, pepper, peppermint, Roman chamomile, rosemary

Stomach, gastralgia or gastritis of
Roman chamomile

Stomach, heartburn and
cardamom, pepper

Stomach, highly acidic
lemon, peppermint

Stomach, infection of
immortelle

Stomach, inflammation of mucous membrane of
lemon, pennyroyal, Roman chamomile

Stomach, tonic for
basil, cardamom, fennel, juniper, lemongrass, Melissa,

myrrh, oregano, pepper, peppermint, Roman chamomile, rose, savory, tangerine, verbena

Stress
See Nerves.

Sunburn
immortelle, lavender, lemon, peppermint, Roman chamomile

Sunstroke
lavender, lemon, Melissa, peppermint, rose

Suprarenal gland, tonic for
fir, geranium, sage

Sweat, inducing
camphor, pennyroyal, peppermint, rosemary, sassafras

Sweat, reducing
See Deodorants.

Syphilis
See Genitals, syphilis affecting.

Teeth, aching
cajeput, clove, nutmeg, pennyroyal, peppermint, Roman chamomile, sage

Teeth and teething
Roman chamomile

Tendonitis
See also Rheumatism.
birch, rosemary

Throat, sore
clary sage, eucalyptus, geranium, lavender

Thrush
myrrh

Tissue, fatty (reducing)
juniper

Tonic, body
basil, cardamom, coriander, fennel, frankincense, geranium, hyssop, jasmine, juniper, lavender, marjoram, Melissa, myrrh, neroli, nutmeg, Roman chamomile, rose, sandalwood

Tonsillitis
bergamot

Tuberculosis
bergamot, camphor, eucalyptus, hyssop, lavender, myrrh

Tumors
cajeput, eucalyptus, tea tree

Typhus
lemon, lavender (fever)

Urinary stones
fennel, geranium, hyssop, juniper, lemon, Roman chamomile

Urinary tract, infection or inflammation of
bergamot, cedarwood, eucalyptus, juniper, lavender, myrrh, myrtle, onion, tea tree, turpentine

Urine, stimulation of secretion of (diuretics)
anise, benzoin, camphor, cardamom, eucalyptus, fennel, garlic, geranium, juniper, lavender, onion, pepper, rosemary, sage

Uterus, tonic for
frankincense, jasmine, Melissa, myrrh, pennyroyal, rose

Vaginal discharge.
See Genitals, vaginal discharge from.

Vaginitis
Roman chamomile, tea tree

Varicose veins
bergamot, cypress, garlic, lemon

Vasoconstrictor (constriction of capillaries)
camphor, cypress, peppermint

Veins, broken
See Skin care, broken veins and.

Viral infections
bergamot, eucalyptus, garlic, tea tree, thyme

Voice, loss of
cypress, lavender, lemon, thyme

Vomiting
basil, lavender, Melissa, peppermint, Roman chamomile, rose, sandalwood

Warts
clove, garlic, lavender, lemon, onion, peppermint, tuja

Weight loss
See Appetite, reducing; Tissue, fatty.

Whooping cough
See Cough, whooping.

Worms
See Intestines, worms in.

Wounds, healing of (formation of scar tissue)
benzoin, bergamot, camphor, clary sage, eucalyptus, frankincense, geranium, hyssop, juniper, lavender, marjoram, myrrh, patchouli, Roman chamomile, rosemary, sage, savory, tea tree

Appendix
Essential Oil Tables
Table 1: Evaporation of Scents at Room Temperature

Fast (evaporates within 3 hours)	Medium (evaporates within 6 hours)	Slow (evaporates within 2 days)
Bergamot	Anise	Amber (Styrax)
Chamomile	Basil	Basil
Eucalyptus	Cardamom	Benzoin
Grapefruit	Clary Sage	Cedarwood
Juniper	Clove	Cinnamon
Lavender	Coriander	Frankincense
Lemon	Cypress	Jasmine
Marjoram	Fennel	Myrrh
Pennyroyal	Geranium	Rose
Rosemary	Hyssop	Sandalwood
Verbena	Niaouli	Vanilla
	Nutmeg	Ylang-ylang
	Orange	
	Pepper	
	Peppermint	
	Petitgrain	
	Pine	
	Sage	
	Tangerine	
	Thyme	

Table 2: Odor Intensity of Essential Oils

Light	Medium	Strong
Benzoin	Anise	Amber (Styrax)
Bergamot	Cajeput	Basil
Camphor	Clary Sage	Cardamom
Cedarwood	Clove	Chamomile
Cypress	Geranium	Cinnamon
Fennel	Ginger	Coriander
Grapefruit	Hyssop	Eucalyptus
Lavender	Juniper	Frankincense
Marjoram	Lemon	Garlic
Myrtle	Lemongrass	Jasmine
Petitgrain	Marjoram	Musk
Pine, Mountain	Neroli	Myrrh
Pine, Stone	Orange	Nutmeg
Rosewood	Oregano	Patchouli
Tangerine	Pennyroyal	Peppermint
	Rose	Vanilla
	Rosemary	Vetiver
	Sage	Ylang-ylang
	Sandalwood	
	Thyme	
	Verbena	

Table 3: Amounts of Essential Oils for Various Blends and Uses

⅛ oz. essential oil equals 70–90 drops
¼ oz. essential oil equals 140–160 drops
½ oz. essential oil equals 280–350 drops
1 oz. essential oil equals 560–700 drops
These amounts are dependent on size of dripper
and consistency of the oil.

Facial Oils: 15–20 drops per 2 oz.
Body Oils: 15–20 drops per 2 oz.
Bath Oils: Up to 50 drops per 2 oz., but use only 1–2
tsp. per bath.
Massage Oils: Up to 25 drops per 2 oz.
Healing Oils for Skin Diseases, Wounds, Inflamma-
tion, Infections, Pimples, Rashes: 60 drops per 2 oz.
Inhalation: Up to 5 drops in up to 2 pints of water.
Compresses: Up to 10 drops in up to 2 pints of water.
Bathing: 6–15 drops.
Aroma Lamp: 6–15 drops.
Internal Use: Maximum 3 drops.
Hair Cure: 6–10 drops.
Hair Rinse: 10 drops in 2 pints of water.
Cleansing Mask: 4–6 drops.

Recommended Reading

For further reading, I suggest the following books:

Cunningham, Scott. *Magical Aromatherapy.* St. Paul, MN: Llewellyn Publications, 1990.

Jackson, Judith. *Scentual Touch.* New York: Fawcett Columbine, 1987.

_____. *The Power of Holistic Aromatherapy.* New York: Javelin Books/Sterling, 1986.

Keller, Erich. *Aromatherapy Handbook for Beauty, Hair, and Skin Care.* New York: Inner Tradition/ Destiny Books, 1991.

Tisserand, Robert B. *The Art of Aromatherapy.* Rochester, VT: Destiny Books, 1977.

Valnet, Jean. *The Practice of Aromatherapy.* Rochester, VT: Destiny Books, 1982.

Erich Keller offers workshops on aromatherapy. He can be reached at the following address:

Erich Keller
Academy of Natural Complementary Medicine
1310 Cibola Circle
Santa Fe, NM 87501

ALSO FROM H J KRAMER INC

THE PERSECUTION AND TRIAL OF GASTON NAESSENS:
*The True Story of the Efforts to Suppress an
Alternative Treatment for Cancer, AIDS, and
Other Immunologically Based Diseases*
by Christopher Bird
A brilliant scientist's heroic struggle against the medical
establishment to apply successful alternative therapies to the
most challenging diseases of today.

EAT FOR HEALTH:
*Fast and Simple Ways of Eliminating
Diseases Without Medical Assistance*
by William Manahan, M.D.
Distinct in the world of health books, this simple guide
gives practical steps for self-diagnosis of food-related illnesses
and how to heal yourself.

AMAZING GRAINS:
Creating Vegetarian Main Dishes with Whole Grains
by Joanne Saltzman
"Makes the process of learning and cooking into what
it is meant to be – a joy."
–John Robbins, author of *Diet for A New America*

ROMANCING THE BEAN:
Essentials for Creating Vegetarian Bean Dishes
by Joanne Saltzman
The companion book to *Amazing Grains* with sixty-six
savory bean recipes for every season.

YOU THE HEALER:
*The World Famous Silva Method on How to
Heal Yourself and Others*
by José Silva and Robert B. Stone, Ph.D.
The complete course in Silva Method healing techniques –
using the power of the mind and alpha frequencies –
in an easy-to-understand forty-day format.

ALSO FROM H J KRAMER INC

WAY OF THE PEACEFUL WARRIOR:
A Book that Changes Lives
by Dan Millman
The international bestseller that speaks directly to the
universal quest for happiness.

THE LAWS OF SPIRIT:
Simple, Powerful Truths for Making Life Work
by Dan Millman
A little book of timeless wisdom – 12 universal principles,
based on the world's great spiritual traditions – for living and
loving well. From the author of *Way of the Peaceful Warrior*.

CREATING MIRACLES:
Understanding the Experience of Divine Intervention
by Carolyn Miller, Ph.D.
The first scientific look at creating miracles in your life.
These simple practices and true stories offer new wisdom
for accessing the miraculous in daily life.

UNDERSTAND YOUR DREAMS:
1500 Dream Images and How to Interpret Them
by Alice Anne Parker
The essential guide to becoming your own dream expert.
This book makes dreaming a pleasure and waking an adventure.

SON RISE:
The Miracle Continues
by Barry Neil Kaufman
Now in paperback! The astonishing real-life account of an
autistic boy's journey from silence to health through the
extraordinary love and commitment of his parents.